MW00682592

Nutritional Medicine pc

Authors:
Elise M. Brett, MD
Associate Clinical Professor
Icahn School of Medicine at Mount Sinai
1192 Park Avenue
New York, NY 10128

Jeffrey I. Mechanick, MD
Clinical Professor
Icahn School of Medicine at Mount Sinai
1192 Park Avenue
New York, NY 10128

Acknowledgements:
Andreas Ruß, MD
Internal Medicine Specialist,
Kirchplatz 1
83734 Hausham

Editing: Dominik Stauber, MD, Bhagyashree Ghugari, MD, Shantanu Patil, MD
Cover Illustration: Mariona Dieguez, Linda Meyer
Production: Alexander Storck
Publisher: Börm Bruckmeier Publishing LLC, www.media4u.com

Printed in China through Colorcraft Ltd., Hong Kong
ISBN 978-1-59103-271-7

Preface

Welcome to the Nutritional Medicine Pocket!

This pocket book was created in response to the increasing importance of nutrition in virtually every aspect of health and medicine. Even as technology and molecular medicine advance, it is the interaction of diet and nutrients from the environment on our metabolism and epigenome that dictate levels of health, expression of disease, and responses to therapy. The book is for physicians, nurses, dietitians, and allied health professionals seeking readily accessible information spanning the breadth of nutrition.

The book was designed for the dietitians and clinicians to be able to find the most relevant and up to date information regarding a particular nutritional problem quickly and easily. It contains pertinent information for treating inpatients and outpatients, with basic and advanced concepts, to be used as needed during hospital rounds or in clinic. Healthy eating, health promotion, and preventive medicine paradigms are detailed as well as specific aspects and treatments for diseases (GI, cancer, obesity, diabetes, critical illness, etc.). Chapters on parenteral and enteral nutrition support are constructed so that the reader can formulate safe interventions and appropriately monitor therapy. A comprehensive section at the end contains numerous tables, lists, and facts that would be difficult to memorize. When needed, clinical trials are cited and relevant references are provided.

We are confident you will find this resource highly valuable in your clinical practice in order to optimize clinical care. If you have any questions or comments, please feel free to contact us at info@media4u.com.

The authors and the publisher   April, 2015

Elise M. Brett, MD   Jeffrey I. Mechanick, MD

1   Diet, Food & Supplements

1.1   Healthy Eating and Conditions

1.1.1   Healthy eating[1, 2]

General principles

- Work on healthy eating patterns
- Adjust calorie intake to achieve or maintain a healthy weight
- Read nutrition facts labels to assist with meal planning
- Limit solid fats, added sugars, and refined grains
- Eat more vegetables, fruits and whole grains and fat free dairy, lean meats, eggs, beans and peas, nuts and seeds, seafood
- Minimize saturated fats; eat healthy fats
- Dietary supplements and nutraceuticals only for proven indications
- Limit sweetened beverages
- Choose nutrient dense foods
- Choose fresh whole foods over processed foods
- Choose foods high in fiber

Macronutrient intake

Calories

See also Determining calorie requirements →194
- Women: 1600-2400 calories/day for weight maintenance
- Men: 2000-3000 calories/day for weight maintenance
- Calorie requirements are at the low end for older age and sedentary lifestyle
- Calorie requirements are typically lower than above ranges for weight loss

Carbohydrates

- Energy source
- Stored as glycogen

Simple	Complex
• Monosaccharides: glucose, fructose, galactose, xylose, ribose • Disaccharides: sucrose, glucose	• Oligosaccharides (3-9 monosaccharides) • Polysaccharides (10+ monosaccharides)

Carbohydrates (cont.)

- Sugar, starches, and fiber
- Provide 4 kcal/g
- Should be 45%-65% of total energy

- 7-12 servings of fruits and vegetables recommended per day
- Fiber intake should be 25-30 g/day

Soluble fiber	Insoluble fiber
- May improve lipids and glycemic control - Eg, oatmeal, oat bran, nuts and seeds, legumes (beans, peas), fruit (apples, blueberries, pears, strawberries)	- Increase stool bulk, help prevent constipation - Eg, whole grain breads and cereals, barley, brown rice, wheat bran, vegetables (carrots, celery, cucumbers, tomatoes, zucchini)

- Choose whole grains over refined grains:
  - Whole grains include the entire kernel
  - Refined grains have been milled to remove the bran and germ to give finer texture and improve shelf life (Food sources of whole grains: wild rice, popcorn, buckwheat, bulgur wheat, millet oatmeal, quinoa, rolled oats, brown or wild rice whole grain barley, brown rice, whole wheat bread, whole grain cereal, whole grain pasta)
  - Most refined grains are enriched with B vitamins and iron
  - Refining results in loss of vitamins, minerals and fiber (Food sources of refined grains: waffles, pancakes, cereals, crackers, potato chips, pasta, tortillas, breads, pizza)

Protein

- Components of muscle, cartilage, ligaments, keratin, nucleic acids, neurotransmitters, hormones, enzymes
- Provides 4 kcal/g
- Composed of amino acids
  - Oligopeptide: 2-20 amino acids
  - Polypeptide: >20 amino acids
  - Protein: polypeptide (usually >40 amino acids) folded into 3 dimensional structure

Amino acids (AA) types

Essential amino acids	Those that are not made in sufficient quantities in the body to prevent disease and must be provided in food eg, arginine, histidine, isoleucine, leucine, lysine, methionine, phenylalanine, threonine, tryptophan, valine

Amino acids (AA) types (cont.)	
Non-essential amino acids	Produced by the body eg, Alanine, asparagine, aspartic acid, cysteine, glutamic acid, glutamine, glycine, hydroxylysine, hydroxyproline, proline, serine, tyrosine
Indispensable amino acids	Those that are not synthesized from ordinarily available precursors at a rate sufficient to meet normal physiological needs, not stored, and rapidly depleted when not provided by the diet eg, lysine and threonine

- Problem with AA categorization:
  - Recent evidence has blurred distinctions between indispensable and dispensable, and essential and nonessential
  - In order to maintain homeostasis, indispensable AA deficiency states must be physiologically sensed
  - Lysine and threonine are totally indispensable amino acids; other carbon-skeleton indispensable amino acids may include leucine, isoleucine, valine, methionine, phenylalanine, tryptophan and possibly histidine)
  - Conditionally or acquired indispensable amino acids: arginine, citrulline, ornithine, cysteine, tyrosine, and possibly taurine
  - Dispensable amino acids: glutamate and serine, possibly aspartate
  - "Conditionally essential" amino acids: Synthesis can occur but is limited by certain factors (dietary supply, age, overall health)
  - Functionally, all AA are considered conditionally essential and the semantic classifications of dispensable and indispensable remain controversial
- Protein should be 10%-35% of total energy
- Protein requirements: 0.8-1.0 g/kg/day:
  - Requirements are higher for stress
  - Requirements are lower for stage IV and V CKD not on renal replacement therapy
- Recommended:
  - 5-6 oz/day of lean meat (1 oz=approx 7 g)
  - 2-3 servings reduced fat dairy (1 serving=8-13 g)
  - Seafood (8 or more oz/week)
- Biological value (BV): The degree to which a protein is absorbed from food and can be incorporated into the body:
  - Higher BV proteins: egg (100), beans (96), cheese (84), beef (80), chicken (79), fish (76)
  - Lower BV proteins: peanuts (55), brown rice (57), tofu (64)
- Preferred sources of animal protein: low-fat dairy (skim milk, reduced fat cheese, yogurt), lean meats, egg whites, fish, skinless poultry
- Sources of plant protein: legumes (beans, lentils) tofu, soy milk, nuts, grains, seeds; plant proteins are typically incomplete (deficient in one or more essential amino acids)

Fat
- Energy source and used in the production of cell membranes, prostaglandins and hormones; Provides 9 kcal/g

Types
- Saturated: eg, palmitic, myristic, stearic, lignoceric
  - Associated with ↑ risk for CAD and ↑ LDL cholesterol
  - Food sources: red meat (beef, pork), high fat dairy products (whole milk, butter, cheese, ice cream), poultry skin, egg yolks, coconut, coconut oil, palm oil, palm kernel oil
- Monounsaturated fatty acids (MUFA): oleic acid
  - Associated with ↓ risk of CAD and ↓ LDL cholesterol
  - Food sources: olive oil, peanut oil, canola oil, avocado, nuts
- Polyunsaturated fatty acids (PUFA)
  - Associated with ↓ risk of CAD, lower LDL cholesterol
  - Liquid at room temperature
  - Omega-6 fatty acids:
    - Linoleic acid: essential FA found in corn oil, safflower oil, sunflower oil
    - Gamma-linolenic acid (GLA): FA found in vegetable oils
  - Omega-3 fatty acids:
    - Alpha-linolenic acid (ALA): essential omega-3 FA found in flaxseed oil, canola oil, soybean oil and nuts (especially walnuts)
  - Other: eciosapentaenoic acid, docosahexaenoic acid found in fish oil (highest content is found in salmon and mackerel)
- Trans fatty acids:
  - Associated with ↑ risk of CAD, high LDL cholesterol
  - Solid at room temperature
  - Produced by heating vegetable oil in the presence of hydrogen
  - Examples include margarine, vegetable shortenings, some French fries, onion rings and baked goods
  - Some natural trans fatty acids occur in meat, milk and milk products
- Triglycerides:
  - Formed by 3 esterified FAs attached to a glycerol backbone
- Fats should be 10%-35% total energy
- Saturated fat intake should be <10% of total daily calories
- Cholesterol intake should be <300 mg/day
- Unsaturated fats (MUFA/PUFA) should be consumed in place of high saturated fat foods
- At least 2 servings of fish per week are recommended
- Processed meats (sausage, bacon, franks) may ↑ risk of CAD and colorectal cancer and should be limited

Micronutrient intake

- Consume 7-12 servings fruit and vegetables daily
- Consume 3 servings reduced-fat dairy per day for calcium eg, fat-free milk, low fat cheese, low fat yogurt, low fat cottage cheese
- Supplementation above RDA not recommended except for vitamin D and deficiency states
- Many people need to supplement vitamin D 800-1000 IU daily
- Older adults should periodically be screened for B12 deficiency

Alcohol

- 7 calories/g
- Mixers contain additional calories
- Limit to 2 drinks per day for men and 1 serving per day for women
  - Beer 12 oz
  - Wine 5 oz
  - Distilled spirits 1.5 oz
- Moderate alcohol consumption is associated with ↓ risk of CVD
- It is not recommended to start drinking for health benefits

Sodium

- <2300 mg/day
- <1500 mg/day for age >50 or hypertension, DM, or CKD
- Consume more fresh foods and fewer processed foods to limit sodium intake

1.1.2   Dyslipidemia

- Mediterranean diet plan:
  - Higher intake: vegetables, fish, nuts, legumes, grains, fish, MUFA
  - Low intake: high fat dairy products, meat, saturated fat
  - ↑ plant protein > animal protein
  - Red wine included in most Mediterranean Diets
  - Meat primarily as fresh fish
  - High in olive oil (high in polyphenols)
  - Cardiovascular benefits thought to be related to dietary fatty acid changes and not LDL or HDL levels
- The therapeutic lifestyle changes meal plan[3]:
  - <7% total calories from saturated fat
  - 25%-35% of total calories from fat
  - <200 mg/day of cholesterol
  - Sodium <2400 mg/day
  - Enough calories to maintain healthy weight

Dyslipidemia (cont.)

- 2-4 servings or fruit per day
- 3-5 servings of vegetables daily
- 6 or more servings of grains per day
- ≤5 oz lean meat daily
- Not more than 2 egg yolks per week

1.1.3   Hypertension

- 10% weight loss for overweight people
- Increased dietary potassium is beneficial if normal kidney function
  - Food sources: bananas, oranges, apricots, avocado, kiwi, artichokes, beets, figs, pears, spinach, prunes, potatoes, orange juice, milk, plain yogurt
- Increase cruciferous vegetables (eg, broccoli, cabbage, cauliflower), lower intake of meat
- DASH meal plan (Dietary Approaches to Stop Hypertension)
  - Results in lower blood pressure and lower risk of CVD
  - High intake of fruit, vegetables, whole grains; reduced intake of fat and dairy
  - Sodium intake <2300 mg
  - Potassium intake >4700 mg
  - Sodium intake <1500 mg/dL for over age 51 or African American
  - ≤5 oz lean meat daily
- Foods that can raise blood pressure
  - Licorice; tyramine containing foods: aged cheese, cured meat, fava beans, smoked meats, sauerkraut, soy sauce, dark beer, red wine

1.1.4   Cardiovascular disease

- Reduce added sugar to <450 kcal/week: avoid sugar sweetened beverages
- Limit sodium to <1500 mg/day
- Limit saturated fat to <7%
- 25%-35% of daily calories as fat
- Limit cholesterol to <200 mg/day
- Enough calories to maintain or lose weight
- Limit processed red meat to <2 servings per week
- Substitute whole grains for refined grains

1.1.5 Diabetes

- Avoid sugar sweetened beverages
- Sucrose does not need to be eliminated for glycemic control:
  - High sucrose foods are often high in saturated fat and total calories
- Protein 15%-30% of total calories (0.8-1.0 g/kg/day)
- Carbohydrate 40%-50% of total calories:
  - Primarily as unprocessed grains, fruits, vegetables
- Fiber 25-30 g/day (14 g/1000 kcal)
- Fat 20%-30% of total calories:
  - Saturated fat <7% of total calories
  - PUFA up to 10% of total calories
  - MUFA up to 15%-20% of total calories
  - Cholesterol <200 mg/day
  - Minimal trans fats
- Sodium <1500 mg/day

Glycemic index

- Glycemic response of various foods are indexed against either 50 g of dextrose or white bread over a standard 120 min time course
  - Accurate only when a food is eaten by itself
  - High GI foods (>70) eg, white bread, doughnut, bagel, cornflakes, pizza, jellybeans, baked potato, French fries, mashed potatoes
  - Low GI foods (<55) eg, legumes, whole oats, dairy, croissant, multigrain bread, ice cream, cashews, yam, mango, apple
- Glycemic load (GL): takes into account the amount of carbohydrate in a food serving
  - Low GL (<10): multigrain bread, apple, lentils, popcorn, beans, pineapple, orange
  - Medium GL (11-19): sweet potato, mashed potato, pizza, salmon sushi, banana, Raisin bran
  - High GL (>20): baked potato, French fries, bagel, cornflakes, macaroni and cheese

1.1.6 Chronic kidney disease

Malnutrition, inflammation, and atherosclerosis syndrome[4]

- 30%-50% of patients with ESRD have evidence of an activated inflammatory response
- Protein-energy malnutrition and wasting due to:
  - Anorexia
  - ↑ resting energy expenditure
  - ↑ muscle protein breakdown
  - Hypoalbuminemia
  - Protein losses through dialysis
- Accelerated atherosclerosis

Protein intake recommendations for stages of CKD

- Stage 1, 2, 3 CKD:
  - Limit protein to 12%-15% of daily intake
  - 0.8 g/kg/day
- Stage 4 and stage 5 CKD not on renal replacement therapy:
  - Reduce to <10% of daily intake
  - 0.6 g/kg/day
- Stage 5 CKD on Renal replacement therapy:
  - Protein 1.3 g/kg/day (peritoneal dialysis)
  - Protein 1.2 g/kg/day (hemodialysis)

Sodium	Limit to <2000 mg/day
Potassium	Limit to 2000-3000 mg/day
Phosphorus	Limit to 800 mg/day in stage 3, 4, 5
Vitamin D	Maintain level of 25-OH vitamin D > 30 ng/mL
Iron	• Maintain ferritin >100 ng/mL • Maintain transferrin saturation >20% • Supplement with iron sulfate 325 mg

1.1.7 Bone health

Calcium intake

- 1000 mg/day for premenopausal women and men
- 1000-1200 mg day for postmenopausal women
- **Food sources**:

>300 mg/serving	• Milk 8oz • Yogurt 6oz	• Fortified orange juice 8 oz
160-249 mg/serving	• Sardines 2 oz • Turnip greens 6 oz • Almonds 3 oz	• Beans 1 cup • Cheese 3 cm cube • Canned salmon
29-159 mg/serving	• Tofu 3 oz • Collard greens ½ cup	• Cottage cheese ¾ cup

- Use supplements if meal plan does not provide sufficient calcium
- Limit to 500-600 mg/dose for adequate absorption
- Individualize therapy in patients with bone loss or history of kidney stones by monitoring 24 h urine calcium
- Use calcium citrate supplements in patient on proton pump inhibitors or H2 blockers

Vitamin D

- Maintain plasma 25-OH vitamin D levels to 30-60 ng/mL
- Daily intake 600-2000 IU for most adults
- Use vitamin D analogs (eg, cholecalciferol [vitamin D3]) in patients with CKD

1.1.8 Pregnancy[5]

- Achieve normal BMI prior to conception
- Macronutrients:
  - Protein 1.1g/kg/day in second and third trimester: Aim for extra 25 g/day of protein
  - <10% fat from saturated fat
  - Avoid trans fats
  - Carbohydrate minimum 175 g/day
- Micronutrients:
  - Daily prenatal vitamin
  - Folate 600 mcg daily: food sources: green leafy vegetables, liver, citrus fruits, juices, fortified grains and cereals
  - Limit vitamin A intake to 10000 IU
  - Calcium 1000 mg/day

Pregnancy (cont.)
- Iron 27 mg/day: food sources: meat, dark poultry, cooked clams and oysters, legumes, enriched grain products
- Iodine 150 mcg/day
- Food sources: iodized salt, milk, fortified bread, cereals, seaweed
- Recommended weight gain:
  - Pre-pregnancy BMI <18.5: 28-40 pounds
  - Pre-pregnancy BMI 18.5-24.9: 25-35 pounds
  - Pre-pregnancy BMI 25-29.9: 15-25 pounds
  - Pre-pregnancy BMI >30: 11-20 pounds
- Recommended weight gain for twins:
  - Pre-pregnancy BMI 18.5-24.9: 37-54 pounds
  - Pre-pregnancy BMI 25-29.9: 31-50 pounds
  - Pre-pregnancy BMI >30: 25-42 pounds
- Consume <300 mg/day caffeine
- All patients should be screened for gestational diabetes
- Foods to eat with caution: unpasteurized dairy (risk of listeriosis) luncheon meats
- Tuna (limit to 6 oz/week)
- Do not eat shark, swordfish, king mackerel, tilefish

1.1.9   Gestational diabetes

- Limit weight gain to 2-5 pounds during first trimester and 0.5-1.0 pound/week thereafter
- Avoid concentrated sweets
- Small frequent meals (3 small meals, 3 snacks)
- Include protein at each meal
- Limit carbohydrates to one serving of starch with breakfast
- Avoid fruit at breakfast
- Choose high fiber foods
- Limit processed foods
- Minimum carbohydrate 175 g/day

1.1.10   Elderly

- ↑ age associated with loss of muscle mass (sarcopenia) and ↓ metabolic rate
- Relatively more high-quality protein is needed eg, lean meat, egg whites, dairy, beans, nuts
- Consider daily multivitamin:
  - Deficiencies in vitamin B12, B6, calcium, iron, and folic acid are more common due to ↓ acid secretion and bacterial overgrowth
- Can also obtain vitamin B12 from fortified cereals
- 3 servings per day of calcium rich foods are recommended
- Avoid dehydration: consume 2 quarts fluid per day
- Nutritional supplements between meals for undernourished
- For carbohydrates, choose whole grains over refined starch
- Include fruits and vegetables
- Limit saturated fat and sugar

1.2   Diets

1.2.1   Diet plans

- Intended as therapeutic or preventive strategies for disease management or health promotion
- Different from dietary patterns, which are retrospective looks at what patients actually eat
- Commercial diets:
  - May or may have proven (scientifically substantiated) benefit
  - Benefits typically short-term and based on limited, often conflicting data
- Consensus diets:
  - Result from scientific evidence
  - Endorsed by professional medical organizations
- Diet plan selection:
  - Based on individual patient factors and discussion with physician
  - Should have proven and relevant long-term benefits with unlikely risks
  - Should be incorporated with physical activity plan

1.2.2   Dietary patterns

- Retrospective look at actual foods and food groups consumed
- Food groupings based on different mathematical models and analytical methods, for example:
  - Fresh fruits and vegetables, whole grains, pulses
  - Food high in saturated fats, red meats
  - Starches and refined sugars
  - Healthy fats, MUFA, ω-3 PUFA, fish, seafood
  - Salty, junk foods
- Can be prospectively correlated with appearance of disease states (diabetes, hypertension, cardiovascular)
- Preferred over commercial diet plans for nutritional counseling
- Healthy dietary patterns:
  - Based on scientifically substantiated commonalities associated with health promotion and disease management
  - Correlated with lower risks for many disease states and complications
  - Serve as basis for consensus diet plans and many commercial diet plans

1.2.3   Commercial diet

Commercial diet*	Type	Rationale	Proven benefit	Potential or proven risks
3-day diet	Balanced	Very-low to low calorie restriction for rapid weight loss	No	Nutrient deficiencies with repeated use
Abs	Balanced	Power foods high in protein, calcium, fiber, healthy fats	No	Unlikely
Atkins	Low-carbohydrate	Calorie restriction and lower insulin promotes lipolysis	Yes	Nutrient deficiencies, low fiber
Biggest loser	Balanced	Calorie restriction, healthy foods, and physical activity	Yes	Unlikely
Cookie	Low-calorie	Scheduled low-calorie snacking to ↓ appetite	No	Unlikely

Commercial diet* (cont.)	Type	Rationale	Proven benefit	Potential or proven risks
Dukan	Low-carbohydrate	Staged diet focusing on high protein and low calories	No	Renal function and bone
Eco-Atkins	Low-carbohydrate	Plant-based version of low-carbohydrate Atkins diet	Yes	Unlikely
Flat belly	Balanced	High in MUFA and based on Mediterranean Diets	Yes	Unlikely
Glycemic index	Balanced	Prioritize GI <55 foods and effects on glycemia	Yes	Unlikely
Jenny Craig	Balanced	Personalized, prepackaged foods, education, fitness	Yes	Unlikely
Macrobiotic	Low-fat	Plant-based, natural, organic, whole foods	Yes	Possible nutrient deficiencies
Master cleanse	Low-calorie	Liquid diet to promote excretion of "toxins"	No	Nutrient deficiencies, organ dysfunction
Mayo clinic	Balanced	Education about healthy eating	Yes	Unlikely
Medi-fast	Low-calorie	Products for 6 meals/day high protein and fiber	Yes	Minor symptoms (cramps, fatigue, etc.)
Mediterranean	Balanced	Pulses, grains, olive oil, fish, MUFA, red wine	Yes	Unlikely
Nutrisystem	Balanced	Prepackaged, delivered, minimal decision-making	Yes	Unlikely

Commercial diet* (cont.)	Type	Rationale	Proven benefit	Potential or proven risks
Opti-fast	Low-calorie	Medically supervised, meal replacement, education	Yes	Unlikely
Ornish	Low-fat	Very low fat, whole grains, aerobics, stress reduction	Yes	Nutrient deficiencies
Paleo	Low-carbohydrate	Avoid refined sugar, dairy, legumes, grains	No	Nutrient deficiencies; saturated fat intake
Pritikin	Low-fat	Very-low fat, low-Na, high-fiber, exercise	Yes	Nutrient deficiencies
Raw food	Low-calorie	↑ consumption of beneficial nutrients	No	Food poisoning
Scarsdale	Low-carbohydrate	Severe carbohydrate reduction for rapid weight loss	No	Porphyria; nutrient deficiencies
Slim-fast	Low-calorie	Use of prepackaged meal/snack replacements	Yes	Unlikely
South beach	Low-carbohydrate	Selection of good carbs and fats, high protein	Yes	Unlikely
Vegan	Balanced	Excludes all animal products including dairy and eggs	Yes	Unlikely
Vegetarian	Balanced	Generally avoids meat, fish, poultry but allows dairy/eggs	Yes	Unlikely
Volumetrics	Balanced	Low-density foods, high fruits/vegetables	Yes	Unlikely

Commercial diet* (cont.)	Type	Rationale	Proven benefit	Potential or proven risks
Weight watchers	Balanced	Point system to motivate selection of healthy foods	Yes	Unlikely
Zone	Balanced	Optimal hormonal/ inflammatory status with 40C/30P/30F	Yes	Unlikely

Consensus diets	Target	Organiz- ations	Rationale	Proven benefit	Potential or proven risks
DASH	Hypertension	NHLBI	High K, Ca, protein, fiber	Yes	Unlikely
Diabetes	Diabetes	ADA, AACE	MNT, low GI, healthy fat	Yes	Unlikely
DGA 2010	Health promotion	IOM, USDA	Plant-based, healthy foods	Yes	Unlikely
Gluten-free	Celiac disease	AGA	↓ gliadin reactions	Yes	Unlikely
Renal	Chronic kidney disease	NKF-K/ DOQI	Focus: protein, micronutrition	Yes	Unlikely
TLC	Cardiovascu- lar disease	NCEP, AHA	Reduced saturated fat	Yes	Unlikely

1.3   Transcultural Nutrition

1.3.1   Diversity in nutrition

- Diversity in nutrition that correlates with different cultures
- New field of study with majority of scientific information based on population studies and case examples; few controlled, interventional studies
- Necessary practice skill to optimize nutritional medical care
- Acculturation: adopting new cultural factors
- Transculturalization: Adapting one dietary strategy (usually evidence based and may be disease-specific) to a specific target culture to improve implementation
- **Examples:**
  - Transcultural diabetes nutrition algorithms for U.S., Asia, Canada, Europe, South America, Persian Gulf
  - Dietary Approaches to Stop Hypertension (DASH) in Korea
- Adaptation of Portuguese version of Subjective Global Assessment for Brazilian patients

Examples of dietary factors in different regions of the world

Asia (rice-based)

Philippines	Relatively low milk intake due to ↑ expense and less availability; ↓ calcium intake as result
Malaysia	Relatively high consumption of sweetened condensed milk and chocolate drinks
Thailand	Decreasing fresh food markets and increasing supermarkets
India	Pulses (eg, dry beans, peas, lentils) are inexpensive protein sources, but are healthy foods; low median protein intake contributes to sarcopenia, insulin resistance, and cardio-metabolic risk, even with relatively lower BMI values
China	Glutinous rice; supplements as part of Chinese medical system
Japan	↑ use of dietary supplements
Singapore	Western-style fast food and ↑ cardio-metabolic risk

Europe (both Western-style and Mediterranean-style)	
Germany	↑ consumption of processed foods, sweets, high-sugar beverages, and cakes
Denmark	More foods from plants, sea and lakes, wild countryside ("New Nordic Diet")
Netherlands	Reconstructing Paleolithic dietary patterns involving macronutrient density and composition, fiber content, electrolyte and pH balance, glycemic load, and omega-3 and -6 fatty acid composition
South and Central America; Caribbean (pediatric obesity problems)	
Mexico	Obesogenic environment is multifactorial; need to focus on stressors and perceptions of corpulence/body image; association of migration to the US and overweight/obesity
Barbados	Childhood obesity focus on tastes for sugary foods and positive parent-child interactions
Persian Gulf (transitional economies and Western-style fast foods with sedentary lifestyle)	

- Vitamin D undernutrition (avoidance of sunlight due to heat) and associations with cardio-metabolic risk factors
- High rate of disordered eating among adolescents

Dietary factors within a particular region of the world

Multi-ethnicities in the U.S.

- Family ecological model can address parents' cultures and behaviors to prevent obesity
- African-Americans: therapeutic diets stress lower fat and higher fresh vegetables in this higher risk population
- Somali refugees: food insecurity with greater intake meat/eggs, lower fruit/vegetables
- Asian-Pacific islanders: selective acculturation with both positive and negative factors in diet and physical activity
- Latinos: health risks due to negative dietary practices from:
  – Acculturation after migration to US
  – Negative dietary practices prior to migration

Native vs. immigrant populations	
General	• Immigrants develop obesity, T2D, and/or CVD with rapid transition to high energy, refined carbohydrate source, and saturated fat with low fiber diet • Immigrants generally in lower socio-economic group
Italy	• Body image differences in immigrants compared with natives
Canada	• Canadian Inuit population: high sugary drink and trans-fat consumption; overweight/obesity • Asians: highest pulse consumption
Maori	Maori are indigenous people of Aotearoa/New Zealand - use of community-derived, culturally-sensitive dietary interventions ("bottom-up") to address ↑ risks, instead of government-dictated "top-down" policy

1.3.2 Prevalence rates in obesity & diabetes

• Highest in Persian Gulf and Middle East
• High in southeast Asia, China, India
• Gender differences:
  – Developing countries: more overweight/obesity in women
  – Developed countries: more overweight/obesity in men

1.3.3 Body composition variations

	Caucasians	Asians
BMI cutoffs		
Overweight	25.0 to 29.9	23.0-25.0 to 24.9-27.4 (depending on region)
Obesity	≥30.0	≥25.0-27.5 (depending on region)
Waist circumference: increased risk		
Male	>40 inches (102 cm)	>90 cm
Female	>35 inches (88 cm)	>80 cm

Sarcopenia

• Increased prevalence in Asians
• Decreased dietary protein intake
• Decreased physical activity, especially resistance training
• Associated with insulin resistance

1.3.4   Other factors

Food supply

- Based on geography: climate, vegetation, coastline
- Infrastructure to process, transport, store, and distribute food
- Indirectly dependent on economics and politics

Religious constraints

- No alcohol and other restrictions in Islamic faith
- Kosher restrictions in Judaism
- Meat and stricter restrictions in Hindu faith
  - India is not a primarily vegetarian nation
  - Jainism: non-violence to all living things - strict veganism

Economics

- Rural versus urban differences within a region
- Wealthy versus poor among nations
- Negative impact of transitional economies

Food politics

- Involvement of government to establish food policy
- South America:
  - Diffusion of food-related transnational corporations
  - Foreign direct investment in food processing
  - Local production of processed food
- North Africa: obesity policy and behavioral change best accomplished via educational programs

Socialization of eating

- Family oriented in Asia, India
- Food-approach behaviors and restrictions by parents influence a child's BMI (eg, more restriction in Black Afro-Caribbean compared with White German families)
- Meals:
  - Lunch is main meal in many European Countries
  - Dinner (lighter meal) in Spain may be after 10-11 pm
- Culinary practices and food preparation
- Healthcare system and training:
  - Physicians may not have nutrition training
  - Variable roles of dietitians for different countries

1.4   Vitamins and Minerals

1.4.1   Definitions and concepts

Essential nutrient	Required for normal physiological function: • Micronutrient: Requirements at levels generally considered <100 mg/day • Macronutrients: Requirements at levels generally considered >100 mg/day • Vitamins, minerals, certain fatty acids, certain amino acids, and water
Vitamin	An organic micronutrient; most are not synthesized in the body
B-complex	The 8 B-vitamins (B1, B2, B3, B5, B6, B7, B9, B12)
Other non-vitamin B-compounds	Gaps in numerical sequence were once thought to be vitamins

Mineral	An inorganic micronutrient:
	• Major minerals: more abundant (required in approximate amounts >100 mg/day)
	• Minor minerals: less abundant (required in approximate amounts ≤100 mg/day)
	  – "Trace elements" (clear role in human physiology)
	  – "Ultra-trace elements" (unclear role in human physiology; required <1 part per million in diet, or 0.050 mg/day)

Dietary reference intakes See also →246	• Recommended Daily Allowance (RDA): average nutrient intake that meets the needs of 97%-98% of healthy people • Adequate Intake (AI): recommended nutrient intake when the RDA is not available • Tolerable Upper Intake Level (TUL): highest safe level of daily nutrient intake • Acceptable Macronutrient Distribution Range (AMDR): Percent intake associated with reduced risk for a particular chronic disease • Vitamins and minerals are generally used for prevention or treatment of deficiency conditions; additional pharmacological uses are included below

Nutrient absorption

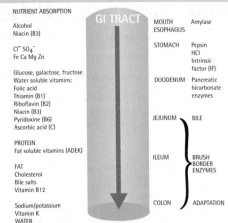

NUTRIENT ABSORPTION

Alcohol	MOUTH	Amylase
Niacin (B3)	ESOPHAGUS	
Cl^- SO_4^-	STOMACH	Pepsin
Fe Ca Mg Zn		HCl
		Intrinsic factor (IF)
Glucose, galactose, fructose		
Water soluble vitamins:	DUODENUM	Pancreatic
Folic acid		bicarbonate
Thiamin (B1)		enzymes
Riboflavin (B2)		
Niacin (B3)		
Pyridoxine (B6)	JEJUNUM	BILE
Ascorbic acid (C)		
PROTEIN		
Fat soluble vitamins (ADEK)	ILEUM	BRUSH BORDER ENZYMES
FAT		
Cholesterol		
Bile salts		
Vitamin B12		
Sodium/potassium	COLON	ADAPTATION
Vitamin K		
WATER		

GI TRACT

1.4.2   Fat soluble vitamins

Vitamin A (retinoids and carotenoids)

Role	Vision, immune function, mucosal integrity, red blood cell production, cellular differentiation, intracellular communication, skin/epithelial tissue
Food sources	Liver, kidney, cream, butter, egg yolk, yellow and green vegetables and fruits
Biochemistry	• 1 IU = 0.3 mcg all-trans retinol • 1 IU = 0.6 mcg all-trans carotene • 1 retinol equivalent (RE) = 1 mcg retinol = 6 mcg β-carotene = 12 mcg other provitamin A carotenoids in foods • Cis forms have about 50% less bioactivity • Function in esterification, oxidation, conjugation, isomerization, and chain cleavage

Vitamin A (cont.)	
	• Binds to transcription factors: retinoic acid receptors (RAR) and retinoid X receptors (RXR)
Absorption, transport, and storage	• Released from protein in stomach during proteolysis • Incorporation into bile salt containing micelle • Bound to retinol-binding protein in plasma • Primarily stored in liver
Deficiency	Poor wound healing, xerophthalmia, keratomalacia, Bitot's spots, blindness, diarrhea
Toxicity	Liver dysfunction, joint pain, bone pain, nausea, headache, osteoporosis; teratogenic

Vitamin D (calciferol; D2: ergocalciferol; D3: cholecalciferol)	
Role	Intestinal absorption of calcium and phosphate; calcium and bone metabolism; immunomodulation
Food sources	Yeast, fish liver oils, fortified milk, fortified margarine: • D2 from phytoplankton, invertebrates, yeasts, higher fungi (can be part of a vegan diet) • D3 occurs naturally in animal skin and milk • Formation of both requires exposure to UV light

Biochemistry	• Synthesized from cholesterol (from 7-dehydrocholesterol by UV light in the skin)
	• Cholecalciferol converted into 25-hydroxyvitamin D (calcifediol; calcidiol), which is measured to assess vitamin D stores; this intermediate is activated by renal 1 α-hydroxylase into 1,25-dihydroxyvitamin D (calcitriol), which binds to the vitamin D receptor
	  – ↑ GI calcium absorption
	  – Mineralization of bone
	  – Renal calcium and phosphate resorption
	  – Cell proliferation and differentiation
	  – Synthesis of neurotropic factors, nitric oxide, glutathione
	• Calcitriol can also be synthesized from monocyte-macrophage 1 α-hydroxylase and then acts as a cytokine
	• Renal 1 α-hydroxylase regulated by calcium, phosphate, fibroblast growth factor 23 (FGF23), and parathyroid hormone (PTH)
	• 1 mcg = 40 international units (IU)

Vitamin D (cont.)	
Absorption, transport, and storage	• Passive and cholesterol-transporter mediated intestinal absorption • Bound in blood by vitamin D binding protein and albumin • Stored in body fat

Vitamin E (tocopherols, tocotrienols)	
Role	Membrane integrity, antioxidant, cell signaling, enzyme activity regulator, transcription factor, inhibits platelet aggregation
Food sources	Vegetable oils, milk, eggs, fish, cereals
Biochemistry	γ-tocopherol is most common tocopherol in diet α-tocopherol is most biologically active form
Absorption, transport, and storage	• Better from foods (eg, cereals) than supplements • Solubilized by bile acids and incorporated into chylomicrons • Taken up by liver and converted into VLDLs and other lipoproteins • Stored in fat
Deficiency	Hemolytic anemia, peripheral neuropathy
Toxicity	Platelet dysfunction, impaired wound healing

Vitamin K (natural: phylloquinone [K1], menaquinone [K2]; synthetic menadione [K3])	
Role	Blood clotting, bone formation
Food sources	Green leafy vegetables, liver
Biochemistry	• Post-translational modification of proteins • Forms γ-carboxyglutamate (Gla) residues - bind calcium • Coagulation: factors VII, IX, X, XI and proteins C, S, Z • Bone: osteocalcin, matrix Gla protein, periostin • Vascular: growth arrest-specific protein 6
Metabolism, absorption, and storage	• Colonic bacteria convert K1 into K2; impaired with small bowel disease, broad-spectrum antibiotics, or in the elderly • Poor absorption • Stored in fat • Continuously recycled in cells - deficiencies are rare
Deficiency	Easy bruising, bleeding, osteoporosis, coronary heart disease
Toxicity	None

1.4.3 Water soluble vitamins

Vitamin B1 (thiamine; thiamin)

Role	Carbohydrate metabolism, thiamin pyrophosphate
Food sources	Pork, beef, liver, eggs, whole > refined grains, brown rice, legumes, yeast extract, sunflower seeds, asparagus, cauliflower, potatoes, oranges
Biochemistry	• Phosphate derivatives function as cofactors in energy and protein metabolism, and biosynthesis of neurotransmitters • Thiamine antagonists in foods: sulfites (preservative), thiaminases (raw fish, shellfish), flavonoids (eg, quercetin), tannic acid (tea), caffeic acid (coffee)
Absorption, transport, and storage	• Cleaved by phosphatases in upper small intestine and absorbed in jejunum and ileum (inhibited by alcohol and folate deficiency) • Low levels - specific carrier-mediated; high levels - passive diffusion • Phosphorylation dependent mucosal uptake and Na+ dependent ATPase dependent release into circulation • Bound to albumin; 90% of total B1 in RBCs • Excreted into urine (↑ with chronic diuretics)
Deficiency	• Optic neuropathy • Wernicke-Korsakoff syndrome:

Wernicke's encephalopathy	**Korsakoff psychosis**
• In susceptible individuals, with/without the acute administration of iv dextrose or parenteral nutrition without B-vitamins • Paralysis of eye movement; abnormal stance, gait, and mental function	• Alcohol amnestic-confabulatory disorder • Cognitive impairment • May have residual permanent features after thiamine repletion

Vitamin B1 (thiamine; thiamin)	

	• Beriberi:
	  – Dry: peripheral neuropathy - symmetric sensory, motor, reflex distal > proximal and calf tenderness
	  – Wet: confusion, muscle atrophy, edema, tachycardia, enlarged heart, CHF and peripheral neuropathy
	  – Infantile: breast-fed by subclinical thiamine-deficient mothers (loud cry, vomit, tachycardia, seizure)
	• Thiamine-responsive megaloblastic anemia; with diabetes and sensorineural deafness
	• Leigh disease: subacute necrotizing encephalomyelopathy; infants
	• Minor forms present with irritability, malaise, confusion, weight loss
	• Deficiency found with malnutrition, thiamine antagonist-rich diet, chronic disease (alcoholism, GI, HIV-AIDS, persistent vomiting, after roux-en-Y bypass bariatric surgery)

Toxicity	None

Vitamin B2 (riboflavin)	
Role	Component of flavin adenine dinucleotide (FAD) and flavin mononucleotide (FMN) coenzymes involved in metabolism; energy metabolism (fat, ketones, carbohydrates, and protein)
Food sources	Fortified cereal, bread, meat, eggs, fish, vegetables, milk
Biochemistry	• Responsible for yellow-orange color in vitamin supplements and the urine after use • Flavoproteins exhibit wide redox potential range, important in electron transport chain • Involved in conversion on folate and pyridoxine into their coenzymes
Absorption, transport, and storage	• Liberated from ingested FAD and FMN molecules by intestinal luminal phosphatases; absorbed in small intestine (carrier-mediated) • Synthesized by colonic flora, especially with fiber-based diet, absorbed in colon (carrier-mediated)
Deficiency	Sore throat, cheilosis (cracked and red lips), angular stomatitis, magenta tongue, seborrheic dermatitis
Toxicity	None

Vitamin B3 (niacin, nicotinic acid)	
Role	Component of NAD and NADH involved in carbohydrate and fat metabolism; DNA repair; steroidogenesis; serotonin synthesis; used therapeutically to raise HDL-cholesterol and lower triglycerides and cardiovascular disease risk
Food sources	Nuts (peanut butter), legumes (beans and peas), whole grains (except maize, which is low in digestible niacin), avocados, dates, tomatoes, leafy vegetables, broccoli, carrots, sweet potatoes, asparagus, mushrooms, tofu, organ meats, chicken, beef, fish (tuna, salmon, halibut), and eggs
Biochemistry	• Synthesized in liver from essential amino acid tryptophan • Niacinamide/nicotinamide has same vitamin activity but no pharmacological activity on lipids • More complex amides and esters also occur • Stimulates G protein-coupled receptor GPR109A, inhibits lipolysis • Stimulates Gi protein-coupled receptor HM74A • Rate-limiting cofactor for histidine decarboxylase (produces histamine) • GPR109A-mediated prostaglandin D2 release from skin Langerhans cells causes flushing (reduced with sustained release niacin, aspirin, ibuprofen, or laropiprant) • Dose-dependent effects: low (15-18 mg/day) - nutritional; intermediate (>50 mg/day) - vasodilation/flushing; high (500 - 3,000 mg/day) - lipid.
Absorption, transport, and storage	• Rapid absorption in the stomach and upper small intestine via SLC67A19 Na-dependent/Cl-independent neutral amino acid transporter • 15%-30% bound to protein in intestine • Stored in limited amounts in the liver • Converted to coenzymes in target tissue

Deficiency	• Pellagra:
	  – Diarrhea
	  – Dermatitis (necklace lesions lower neck, hyperpigmentation, thick skin, red, scaly rash, sensitivity to sunlight)
	  – Dementia, delirium, amnesia
	  – Stomatitis and glossitis
	  – Death if untreated

Vitamin B3 (cont.)

- Mild deficiency:
  - Metabolism is decreased
  - Cold intolerance
  - Irritability, anxiety, restlessness
  - Poor concentration
  - Fatigue, apathy, depression
- Secondary deficiencies:
  - Carcinoid: Metabolic diversion of niacin precursor to serotonin
  - Hartnup's disease: impaired intestinal absorption/renal resorption of tryptophan

Vitamin B5 (pantothenic acid)	
Role	Component of coenzyme A involved in acetylation reactions (intracellular carbon transport); biosynthesis of proteins, carbohydrates, and fats; signal transduction; enzyme activation/deactivation
Food sources	Nearly ubiquitous in food - meat, liver, kidney, yeast, eggs, broccoli, fish, chicken, milk, avocado, broccoli, yogurt, whole grains
Biochemistry	• Synthesized by microorganisms from pantoic acid and -alanine • Pyruvate enters Krebs cycle as acetyl CoA • α-ketoglutarate converted into succinyl-CoA
Absorption, transport, and storage	• Intestinal luminal conversion of CoA and acyl carrier protein (ACP) in food into free pantothenic acid (hydrolysis and dephosphorylation) • Saturable, Na-dependent active transport • Some passive absorption with high ingested levels • Transported as bound forms in erythrocytes • Hormonal (insulin, glucocorticoids, thyroid hormone) control of tissue levels; pantothenate kinase is rate-limiting step in CoA synthesis in cytosol; enters mitochondria by specific transporter • CoA levels affected by alcohol, B12, Reyes syndrome, starvation, diabetes, certain tumors, steroids, insulin, glucagon, clofibrate • Urinary excretion

Vitamin B5 (cont.)	
Deficiency	• Impaired acetylcholine synthesis: numbness, tingling, muscle cramps • ↓ energy, restlessness, irritability, fatigue, apathy • Hypoglycemia due to ↑ insulin receptor sensitivity (↓ acetylation by palmitic acid) • Other effects: adrenal insufficiency, hepatic encephalopathy, nausea/vomiting, abdominal cramps, abnormal sleep
Toxicity	None

Vitamin B6 (pyridoxine, pyridoxal, pyridoxamine)	
Role	Component of pyridoxal phosphate required for transamination and decarboxylation; Na/K balance; erythropoiesis; monoamine neurotransmitter synthesis (serotonin and catecholamines)
Food sources	Wheat, corn, meat, liver
Biochemistry	• Converted to biologically active pyridoxal-5'-phosphate (P5P) • Can decrease homocysteine • Cofactor for amino acid decarboxylase • Transamination of amino acids to keto-acids (for fuel) • Glycogen cleavage • Formation of δ-aminolevulinic acid (heme precursor) • Phosphatidylserine decarboxylation to phosphatidylethanol-amine (phospholipid synthesis) • Side-chain cleavage cofactor
Absorption, transport, and storage	• Absorbed in upper small intestine via simple diffusion • Transported to liver for conversion into P5P, which is exported bound to albumin • Tissue uptake after extracellular dephosphorylation and then intracellular metabolic trapping as P5P
Deficiency	Irritability, confusion, depression, anemia, neuropathy, seizure, rash, stomatitis
Toxicity	Sensory neuropathy, impaired coordination, fatigue

Vitamin B7 (biotin; vitamin H; coenzyme R)	
Role	Transfers CO_2, synthesis of fatty acids, isoleucine/valine catabolism; gluconeogenesis and Krebs cycle; cell growth
Food sources	• As biocytin, protein-bound • Swiss chard, liver, leafy greens, peanuts, corn • Raw egg yolk; but raw egg whites contain the protein avidin, which tightly binds to biotin and reduces biotin bioavailability • Bioavailability from foods depends on body's ability to break biotin-protein bonds

Biochemistry	• Synthesized from alanine and pimeloyl-CoA
	• Coenzyme for carboxylase enzymes (CO_2 transfer)
	  – Acetyl CoA carboxylase - α, -β
	  – Methylcrotonyl CoA carboxylase
	  – Propionyl CoA carboxylase
	  – Pyruvate carboxylase
	• Biotinylation requires ATP, holocarboxylase synthetase, and covalently attaches to -amino group of lysine residues
	• Biotinidase biotinylates histone proteins

Absorption, transport, and storage	• Intestinal microflora biotin production > metabolic needs of body • Dietary biotin converted to free biotin prior to absorption in small and large intestine • Saturable, Na-dependent, carrier-mediated shared with vitamin B5 and lipoate (human sodium-dependent multivitamin transporter; hSMVT) • Free and bound forms in plasma • Tissue uptake by hSMVT
Deficiency	• Rare, due to intestinal microflora production: no recommended intake amounts • Holocarboxylase synthetase enzyme (covalently links biotin to carboxylase), or biotinidase deficiencies can induce biotin deficiency • Low levels with chronic alcoholism, partial gastrectomy, achlorhydria, burn, seizure disorder, aging, athletics, smoking, or >2 raw eggs daily for months • ↑ demand with pregnancy and lactation (deficiency associated with congenital malformations: cleft palate)

Vitamin B7 (cont.)	
	• Symptoms: hair loss, achromotrichia, perosis, fatty liver, conjunctivitis, dermatitis (scaly red rash around eyes, nose, mouth, genitalia), depression, lethargy, ↓ appetite, paresthesia, hallucination, impaired immunity, abnormal fat distribution • ↑ 3-hydroxyisovaleric acid, ketolactic acidosis, organic aciduria, hyperammonemia
Toxicity	None

Vitamin B9 (folate, folic acid; vitamin M/Bc)	
Role	Coenzyme for transferring single carbon units for attachment in many reactions, DNA synthesis, methylation, and repair; erythropoiesis, male and female fertility
Food sources	Liver, yeast, green leafy vegetables, legumes; fortified cereals and breads

Biochemistry	• Folic acid needs to be converted to tetrahydrofolate (THF) for bioactivity
	• Deficiency leads to homocysteine accumulation
	• Some anti-cancer drugs target folate metabolism and action
	  – Methotrexate conversion of dihydrofolate to THF
	  – Leucovorin (folinic acid; formyl THF) reverse methotrexate toxicity

Absorption, transport, and storage	• Absorption in proximal > distal jejunum > ileum
	• Transmembrane binders
	  – Reduced folate carrier (RFC) - saturable, inactive below pH 6.5
	  – Protein coupled folate transporter (PCFT) - nearly inactive at pH 7.4, small intestine absorption, kidney, liver, placenta, brain
	  – ATP binding cassette exporter (multidrug resistance-associated protein [MRP 1-4])
	  – Mitochondrial folate transporter
	  – Lysosomal folate transporter
	  – Folate binding proteins (receptors, high-affinity [-α, -β, γ-])
	• Transport:
	  – Uptake by liver from portal circulation, metabolized into polyglutamates or released into blood/bile; some enterohepatic circulation
	  – Low-affinity protein binders (albumin)
	  – Soluble folate receptors
	  – RBC folate (marker of long-term status)
	  – 500-20,000 mcg in stores (takes months for deficiency state to appear without folate in diet)

Vitamin B9 (cont.)	
Deficiency	• Macrocytic anemia, neural tube defects, diarrhea, peripheral neuropathy, cognitive and behavioral changes, glossitis, stomatitis, headache, palpitations • B12 deficiency induces secondary folate deficiency
Toxicity	High folic acid dosing masks diagnosis of B12 deficiency
Vitamin B12 (Cobalamin)	
Role	Methylation (homocysteine to methionine and methylmalonyl CoA to succinyl CoA); neurological/hematological function; DNA synthesis; fatty acid and energy metabolism
Food sources	Liver, kidney, meat, milk, egg (↑ bioavailability with cooking), cheese, fish, shellfish
Biochemistry	• Only bacteria can synthesize • Contains cobalt (therefore, no independent requirement for elemental cobalt) • Regenerates folate • Cofactor for isomerases, methyltransferases, and dehalogenases due to reactive carbon–cobalt bond • 5'-deoxyadenosylcobalamin: cofactor of methylmalonyl CoA mutase (elevated methylmalonic acid is a marker of B12 deficiency) • Methylcobalamin: cofactor of 5-methyltetrahydrofolate-homocysteine methyltransferase (elevated homocysteine observed with B12 deficiency) • Cyanocobalamin: main form in foods and supplements; trace amounts of cyanide liberated with metabolism; worse with smoking • Hydroxycobalamin: used with thiosulfate for cyanide poisoning
Absorption, transport, and storage	• Consumed in food bound to protein; liberated by gastric acid and digestive enzymes (pepsin) • Free B12 then binds with R-proteins, produced by salivary glands (prevents degradation in acidic stomach) • Duodenal proteases liberate B12 again, which then binds in-trinsic factor, produced by gastric parietal cells in response to food, histamine, and gastrin (prevents degradation by intestinal bacteria) • Absorption of IF/B12 via terminal ileum receptors and enters portal circulation

Vitamin B12 (cont.)	
	• B12 transfers to transcobalamin II for plasma transport and binding to target cell receptors
	• 2-5 mg stored (50% in liver) with only 0.1% lost daily due to efficiency enterohepatic circulation (> 1-2 years worth stored)
Deficiency	• Macrocytic anemia, gait disturbance, paresthesia, memory loss, fatigue, depression
	• Risks: alcohol use, pernicious anemia (autoimmune destruction of gastric parietal cells and insufficient intrinsic factor production), Crohn's disease involving terminal ileum, and various drugs (eg, metformin, phenytoin, and proton pump inhibitors)
	• Treatment can unmask polycythemia vera, provoke hypokalemia or gout, and mask folate deficiency
Toxicity	None

Choline	
Role	Precursor for acetylcholine; cell membranes structure and physiology; source for methyl groups
Food sources	Egg, fatty meats, liver, cod fish, chicken, dairy, soybean, cauliflower, spinach, wheat germ, kidney beans, quinoa, amaranth
Biochemistry	• In phospholipids: phosphatidylcholine and sphingomyelin
	• Contributes methyl group via betaine and S-adenosylmethionine (SAMe) synthesis
Absorption & transport	• Ingested choline freed by pancreatic enzymes and then absorbed in upper intestine or transformed by bacteria into trimethylamine
	• Free choline taken up by liver via portal circulation; lipid-bound choline enters lymphatics and bypasses liver
	• Distributed to all tissues via lipoproteins (phosphatidylcholine in VLDL particles)
	• Enters target tissue via Na-dependent high and low affinity uptake and other unique transporters
	• Stored as membrane bound phosphatidylcholine
Deficiency	• Risks: vegetarians, vegans, athletes, alcohol use
	• Undernutrition prevalent
	• Elevated ALT, homocysteine,
	• Neural tube defects (↑ requirement with pregnancy)
Toxicity	Fishy smell (trimethylamine), nausea, vomiting, hypotension, sweating, salivation, diarrhea, depression, seizure

Vitamin C (ascorbic acid)

Role	Collagen synthesis, wound healing, prevent capillary bleeding, antioxidant, electron donor
Food sources	Citrus fruits, berries, green and red chili peppers, green leafy vegetables, tomatoes, potatoes, liver, oysters; cooking reduces vitamin C content as much as 60%
Biochemistry	• Glutathione maintains vitamin C in a reduced state (to donate electrons) • Synthesis of collagen, carnitine, neurotransmitters via dopamine β hydroxylase • Peptide amidation for stability • Tyrosine metabolism • ↓ histamine release and detoxification
Absorption, transport, and storage	• Active transport: Na-ascorbate cotransporters (SVCT1/2) and hexose transporters (GLUT1/3); dietary sugar slows absorption • Simple diffusion • Fractional absorption ranges 33% (high intake) to 98% (low intake) • Transported in free form to organs and rapidly excreted with high levels (half-life 30 min) and stored longer with deficiency states (half-life up to 83 days); stores depleted in 1-6 months depending on initial status • Concentrated in certain tissues: adrenal, pituitary, thymus, corpus luteum, retina > brain, spleen, lung, lymph nodes, intestinal mucosa, WBC, pancreas, kidney, salivary glands • Renal excretion or oxidation by L-ascorbate oxidase
Deficiency	• Scurvy: – Brown spots on skin over thighs and legs – Joint pain and swelling – Follicular keratosis – Spongy gums – Bleeding from mucous membranes – Open, suppurating wounds – Loss of hair and teeth – Fatigue

1.4.4   Major minerals

Calcium

Role	Essential for cell signaling, bone health, exocytosis, muscle contraction, cardiac electrical conduction, enzyme cofactors (clotting)
Food sources	Dairy, eggs, canned fish with bones, green leafy vegetables, nuts, seeds, soybeans, tofu, thyme, oregano, dill, cinnamon, figs, quinoa, okra, broccoli, seaweed
Biochemistry	Ionized calcium is bioavailable form

Absorption, transport, and storage	• Gastric acid stabilized free calcium in presence of dietary phosphate
	• Absorption in duodenum:
	  – Low intake via transporter: transient receptor potential cation channel - TRPV6; associated with vitamin D-dependent calcium-binding protein - calbindin
	  – High-intake via passive diffusion; independent of vitamin D
	  – Food: 15%–40% and decreases with aging; fruits and vegetables may reduce absorption but also reduce urinary excretion (no net effect)
	  – As carbonate (oyster shell): 40% calcium; 10% absorbed
	  – As tribasic phosphate: 39% calcium; 10% absorbed
	  – As lactate (dairy): 37% calcium; 33% absorbed
	  – As citrate: 21% calcium; 50% absorbed
	  – As ionic (coral): 100% calcium; 98% absorbed
	• Transported in blood bound to protein or free (ionized)
	• Stored in bones (99% total stores) and teeth
	• Elimination in urine, feces, and sweat

Deficiency	• Risks:
	  – Lactose-intolerance: non Indo-European descent
	  – Vegans: avoidance of dairy
	  – High dietary oxalate: spinach, rhubarb, almonds, cashews, beets
	  – High sodium and protein intake: ↑ urinary excretion
	  – Milk allergy
	• Mechanisms:
	  – Decreased absorption: GI disease, vitamin D deficiency, medications (antacids), pancreatitis, high dietary phosphate, alcohol
	  – Hypoparathyroidism; Malnutrition and eating disorders

Calcium (cont.)	

	• Symptoms:
	  – CATS: convulsions, arrhythmias, tetany, spasms
	  – Petechiae, laryngospasm
	  – Trousseau's and Chvostek's signs

Toxicity	Hypercalcemia (nausea, vomiting, anorexia, thirst, constipation, abdominal pain, weakness, myalgia, confusion, lethargy), hypercalciuria, renal stones, milk-alkali syndrome, ↓ drug absorption

Chlorine	
Role	Major extracellular anion; osmotically active; acid-base status
Food sources	Table salt
Biochemistry	• Bicarbonate-chloride exchange (chloride shift) • Chloride transporters and channels
Absorption, transport, and storage	• Active and passive absorption in small intestine • Sodium-proton-chloride-bicarbonate exchangers in colon • Cystic fibrosis transmembrane conductance regulator (CFTR); ABC transporter across epithelial cell membranes • Congenital chloridorrhea: abnormal transport in ileum • Excretion in urine, feces, and sweat
Deficiency	• Excess loss in gastric secretions with protracted vomiting • Limits bicarbonate excretion • Hypochloremic alkalosis • Sodium resorption
Toxicity	Metabolic acidosis

Magnesium	
Role	Interacts with pyrophosphate compounds (ATP), nucleic acids (genomic stability and DNA repair), enzyme activator, cell signaling (regulates calcium and potassium channels)
Food sources	Cashews, almonds, soybeans, cocoa (dark chocolate), spinach, chard, sea vegetables, tomato, halibut, beans, ginger, cumin, cloves, bran, cereals, coffee

Biochemistry	• Occurs as Mg^{2+} ion • Intracellular levels related to intracellular potassium • Binds to cell membranes • Mg^{2+} transporter complex interacts with tightly bound hydration shells of the ion
Absorption, transport, and storage	• 20%–50% absorption from food • Intracellular diffusion, solvent drag, and active transport in distal small intestine • Negligible saturable component in descending colon with low intake • Vitamin D dependent and independent absorption • Binds weakly to proteins • 60% stored in bones; 20% stored in muscle • 99% intracellular • Primary renal excretion (↑ with vitamin D)
Deficiency	• ↓ absorption with low and high protein intake; GI disease • Phytates, phosphate, and fat ↓ absorption • Seen with alcoholism and diuretics • Renal Mg^{2+} wasting (Bartter's, Gitelman's syndromes) • Symptoms: muscle spasms, bone loss, arrhythmia, hypertension, insomnia
Toxicity	Diarrhea

Phosphorus

Role	Component of DNA, RNA, ATP, and membrane phospholipids
Food sources	Primarily from protein sources such as red meat, dairy, fish, poultry, bread, rice, oats
Biochemistry	• High-energy bonds • Buffering agent • Crystalline calcium-phosphate: hydroxyapatite • Tooth enamel: fluoroapatite

Phosphorus (cont.)	
Absorption, transport, and storage	• Passive and active transport in duodenum • Vitamin D - dependent Na-Pi cotransport • Other mechanisms: vitamin D independent; thyroid and glucocorticoid modulation • Only 1% circulates in blood • 85%-90% stored in bones and teeth as apatite; 70% organic and 30% inorganic forms • Renal excretion; as phosphate ions
Deficiency	• Malnutrition, malabsorption, metabolic syndromes (refeeding), renal wasting, vitamin D deficiency, respiratory alkalosis, alcoholism • Myopathy, neuropathy
Toxicity	Diarrhea, ectopic calcification; impaired Fe, Ca, Mg, Zn utilization
Potassium	
Role	Neurological function, osmotic regulation, muscle contraction
Food sources	Legumes, potato skin, tomato, banana, papaya, pulses, spinach, turmeric, parsley, dried apricots, chocolate, almonds, pistachios, avocados, soybeans, bran
Biochemistry	Na^+/K^+-ATPase pump for cell membrane electrochemical gradient (3 Na^+ out and 2 K^+ in)
Absorption, transport, and storage	• 90% absorption; small intestine; passive • Intracellular cation • Obligatory renal excretion; minor excretion in sweat
Deficiency	• Results from vomiting, diarrhea, renal losses (wasting, mineral-corticoids, diuretics), redistribution (insulinization, refeeding) • Weakness, ileus, EKG changes, alkalosis, arrhythmia, respiratory failure
Toxicity	EKG changes/palpitations, malaise, weakness, sudden death; seen with primary adrenal insufficiency
Sulfur	
Role	Amino acids, peptides, protein, enzymes; electron shuttles, collagen synthesis
Food sources	Eggs, dairy, meat, seafood, nuts, seeds, durian, garlic, onions, asparagus, cabbage, brussels sprouts, broccoli, kale, turnips

Sulfur (cont.)	
Biochemistry	• Antioxidant or reducing agent; oxidizes carbon to create negative charge in organosulfur compounds; reduces oxygen • Part of antioxidants: glutathione and thioredoxin • Part of amino acids: cysteine and methionine (incorporated in protein), homocysteine and taurine (not incorporated into protein) • Cystine is the dimeric amino acid composed of two cysteine molecules joined by disulfide bond • Confers strength to protein keratin in skin and hair • Biotin and thiamine contain sulfur • Metalloproteins: complexes with iron, copper, nickel • Hepatic detoxification of drugs
Absorption, transport, and storage	• Absorption of methionine and cysteine • 20% of dietary methionine is transmethylated to homocysteine, and trans-sulfurated to cysteine (associated with gut mucosal integrity/inflammation, formation of polyamines and S-adenosylmethionine, epigenetic DNA methylation, and colon carcinogenesis) • Sulfate transporters: NaSi-1 and sat-1 (renal), DTDST, DRA (intestinal), AE1 (RBC) • Excretion in bile and urine
Deficiency	Fatigue, brittle nails and hair, arthritis, rash, fat maldigestion, allergies
Toxicity	None
Sodium	
Role	Circulatory volume and blood pressure, osmotic and pH balance, neuronal function, membrane function, signal transduction
Food sources	Table salt, sea vegetables, milk, spinach
Biochemistry	• Sodium channels: voltage- or ligand- gated • Na^+/K^+-ATPase antiporter enzyme

Absorption, transport, and storage	• Active: 20% independent; 80% dependent (eg, cotransport with glucose, amino acid, bile acid, chloride [carrier-; electrical-coupling])
	  – Jejunum: cotransport
	  – Ileum: independent; against electrochemical gradient
	  – Colon
	• Passive

Sodium (cont.)	
Deficiency	• Volume depletion, indirect hyponatremia via ↑ ADH; exercise-induced • Nausea/vomiting, headache, confusion, lethargy, fatigue, coma, anorexia, irritability, weakness, muscle spasm, cramps, seizure
Toxicity	Hypertension

1.4.5 Trace elements

Chromium	
Role	Insulin signaling
Food sources	Processed meats, whole grains, broccoli, green beans, beef, liver, eggs, chicken, oysters, wheat germ, green peppers, apples, bananas, spinach, coffee, nuts, spices
Biochemistry	• Biologically relevant form: trivalent Cr^{3+} • Insulin-mediated chromic ion flux into cell • Binds chromodulin oligopeptide, complex binds insulin receptor-subunit, then increases insulin receptor autophosphorylation via tyrosine kinase • Activation of membrane phosphotyrosine phosphatase
Absorption, transport, and storage	• 0.5%-2% absorbed in small intestine, inversely related to intake • ↑ absorption with amino acids, vitamin C, niacin • Transported to insulin-sensitive cells by transferrin (only 30% loaded with iron) and albumin • Accumulates in liver, bone, spleen • Urinary excretion ↑ with dietary simple sugars • 98% excreted in feces
Deficiency	Impaired glucose tolerance, hyperglycemia, hypertriglyceridemia, peripheral neuropathy, weight loss, confusion
Toxicity	Acute toxicity rare; kidney failure, liver failure with chronic high doses

Copper	
Role	Wound healing, antioxidant, insulin receptor signaling
Food sources	Organ meats, cashews, walnuts, seeds, shellfish, chocolate, mushrooms, spinach, greens, tempeh, barley
Deficiency	Pancytopenia, ↑ LDL, reduced glucose tolerance, cardiomyopathy
Toxicity	Liver failure, kidney failure

Iodine	
Role	Thyroid hormone biosynthesis
Food sources	Seaweed, cod, iodized salt, baked potato, milk, shrimp, turkey, navy beans, tuna, egg
Biochemistry	• Iodine is a diatomic molecule consisting of two iodides interacting via weak van der Walls forces • Organification of iodide with tyrosine residues from thyroglobulin, mediated by thyroid peroxidase, producing thyroid hormones: thyroxine (T4) and triiodothyronine (T3) • Thyroid gland needs 70 mcg/day to produce sufficient thyroid hormone
Absorption, transport, and storage	• Absorbed in small intestine via Na-iodide symporter (reduced with high iodine diet) • Inorganic iodine completely absorbed • Organic iodine incompletely reabsorbed as part of entero-hepatic circulation of thyroid hormones; ↓ with dietary soy • Concentrated in thyroid >> ovaries, skin, salivary glands, breasts, stomach
Deficiency	• Hypothyroidism: goiter, fatigue, cognitive dysfunction, depression, weight gain, low body temperature • Low dietary iodine in inland areas with little seafood • Other risk factors: pregnancy, radiation exposure, goitrogen ingestion, smoking
Toxicity	Worse with selenium deficiency; can be lethal at 30 mg/kg
Iron	
Role	Heme biosynthesis and oxygen transport; energy metabolism
Food sources	Red meat, whole and enriched grains, dry beans and fruit, eggs, spinach, chard, turmeric, cumin, parsley, lentils, tofu, asparagus, salad greens, soybeans, shrimp, fish, beans, tomato, olives
Biochemistry	• Ferrous (Fe^{2+}); ferric (Fe^{3+}) • Electron donor and acceptor • Bound to proteins to prevent unregulated free radical formation • Oxidative phosphorylation, electron transport, redox reactions (cytochromes) • Iron-sulfur proteins

Iron (cont.)	
Absorption, transport, and storage	• Highly regulated steps to optimally conserve iron • Gastric acid lowers pH and rapidly oxidizes and then solubilizes iron • 5%–35% absorbed in duodenum; best with animal products • Absorbed as part of heme or free form through different mechanisms • Ferrous absorbed by divalent metal transporter-1 (DMT1) • Ferric form converted to ferrous form by duodenal cytochrome b reductase (Dcytb) • Absorption ↑ with ascorbate, citrate, amino acids, and iron deficiency • Absorption ↓ with phytates, tannins, soil clay, iron overload, antacids or via competitors: lead, cobalt, strontium, manganese, zinc • Enterocytes can store iron in ferric form bound to apoferritin, sloughed off to feces or moved into body by ferroportin, coregulation by hephaestin (ferroxidase; conversion ferrous to ferric) and hepcidin (master regulator; hepatic peptide) • Circulates bound to transferrin • Ferroportin distributed throughout body and regulates iron stores • Recycling of RBC and conservation of iron by reticulo-endothelial system • 4-5 g stores: about 2.5 g as hemoglobin, 2 g as ferritin complexes, primarily in bone marrow, liver, spleen • Small losses through skin and GI mucosa shedding (1 mg/day males; 1.5-2 mg/day females) • Increased losses with menstruation, pregnancy, lactation
Deficiency	• Early subtle non-specific symptoms with decreasing stores: fatigue • Iron-deficiency anemia • Organ dysfunction and death once oxygen transport significantly impaired • Risks: Increased demand, inflammation (hepcidin-mediated), GI disease (Crohn's, celiac), dietary, inhibition of absorption by phytates (inositol hexokisphosphate; bran/seeds), calcium, tannins (eg, black tea)
Toxicity	Iron overload, hemochromatosis, hepatopathy, cardiomyopathy

Manganese	
Role	Enzyme cofactor; brain function
Food sources	Pineapple, nuts, wheat germ, spelt, brown rice, tempeh, rye, soybeans, tea, spinach, pineapple, thyme, berries, garlic, squash, eggplant, cloves, cinnamon, turmeric
Biochemistry	• Cofactor for oxidoreductases, transferases, hydrolases, lyases, isomerases, ligases, lectins, integrins • Polypeptides containing Mn: arginase (required for ammonia clearance) and superoxide dismutase (Mn-SOD; free radical scavenging)
Absorption, transport, and storage	• 3%–5% dietary Mn is absorbed in intestine; affected by carbohydrate source, phytates, animal protein, other minerals (eg, absorption inhibited by iron, calcium, and magnesium) • Transporters: divalent metal transporter-1 (DMT1), ZIP-8 (zinc transporter), transferrin receptor, voltage-regulated and store-operated Ca^{2+} channels, and ionotropic glutamate receptor Ca^{2+} channels • Crosses blood-brain barrier by active transport and facilitated diffusion • Stored primarily in bones, liver, kidneys • Bound to metalloproteins (eg, glutamine synthetase) in brain • Absorbed Mn excreted in bile (nonabsorbed Mn appears in feces)
Deficiency	Glucose intolerance, skin rash, bone demineralization
Toxicity	Seizure, abnormal bone formation, neurodegenerative disease (impaired speech, bradykinesia, gait disturbance; motor dysfunction syndrome: "manganism"), ↑ risk with hepatopathy
Molybdenum	
Role	Component in enzymes; protein synthesis, purine catabolism, growth; nitrogen, sulfur, and carbon cycles
Food sources	Pork, lamb, beef liver, legumes, lentils, grains, tomatoes, cucumbers, onions, carrots, green beans, eggs, sunflower seeds, wheat flour
Biochemistry	• Metal at enzyme active site: xanthine oxidase (oxidizes xanthine to uric acid), sulfite oxidase, aldehyde oxidase • Forms compounds with carbohydrates and amino acids

Molybdenum (cont.)	
Absorption, transport, and storage	• 50%–93% absorbed in intestine (more as liquid food source, less as solid food source) • Rapid turnover compartment (intestine) and slow turnover compartment (liver) • Transported as a molybdate (MoO_4^{2-}) • Highest concentrations in liver and kidneys • Dietary tungsten reduces molybdenum concentrations • Renal excretion
Deficiency	• Risks: low soil concentrations, parenteral nutrition (without molybdenum) • High serum sulfite and urate • Possible association with certain cancers
Toxicity	Possible gout, possible neurologic symptoms, diarrhea, growth retardation, infertility, copper deficiency
Selenium	
Role	Antioxidant, thyroid hormone metabolism
Food sources	Brazil nuts, bread, cereal, barley, cheese, lamb, mushrooms, cold water fish, tuna, eggs, mustard, garlic, tofu, seeds, dairy
Biochemistry	• Component of glutathione peroxidase, iodothyronine deiodinases, thioredoxin reductase (involved in thyroid hormone metabolism), and the amino acids selenocysteine and selenomethionine • Selenide is metabolic intermediate
Absorption and transport	• Intestinal amino acid transporters and SLC26 multifunctional anion exchanger for selenite • Selenoprotein P is major circulating transport form • Receptor-mediated tissue selenoprotein P uptake • Megalin (low density lipoprotein 2; Lrp2) mediates selenoprotein P uptake from glomerular filtrate
Deficiency	• Risks: Severe intestinal disease, parenteral nutrition (without selenium), advanced age, selenium-deficient soil, high mercury exposure, vitamin E deficiency • Impaired immune function, cardiomyopathy (Keshan disease), possibly osteochondropathy (Kashin-Beck disease)
Toxicity	Selenosis: garlic odor, alopecia, dystrophic fingernails, nausea, diarrhea, fatigue, neurological impairment, cirrhosis, pulmonary edema, death

Zinc	
Role	Enzyme function, transcription factors, wound healing, carbohydrate metabolism, signal transduction, regulates apoptosis, brain function, immunity
Food sources	Oysters, lobster, scallops, beef, veal, pork, lamb, calf liver, eggs, dried beans, seeds, nuts, mushrooms, spinach, asparagus, green peas, yogurt, oats, miso
Biochemistry	• Interacts with organic molecules; binds to amino acid side chains (aspartic acid, glutamic acid, cysteine, histidine) • Flexible coordination geometry allowing different protein conformations • Carbonic anhydrase for CO_2 regulation • Carboxypeptidase cleaves peptide linkages • Zinc fingers, twists, and clusters in transcription factors
Absorption, transport and storage	• Released from food during digestion, then bound to secreted ligands to be absorbed in duodenum and jejunum • Transport proteins and passive diffusion • Intestinal metallothionein modulates absorption by 15%-40% • High iron/copper reduces zinc absorption; high zinc reduces iron/copper absorption (metals compete for metallothionein absorption) • In serum, bound to albumin > transferrin • Concentrates in prostate, eye, prostate, brain, muscle, bones, kidney, liver • Stored in metallothionein reserves in liver or intestinal flora • Losses in urine, skin, bile/feces (enterohepatic circulation)
Deficiency	• Risks: malabsorption, dietary phytates, chronic liver or kidney disease, sickle cell, diabetes, cancer, other chronic diseases • Symptoms/signs: scaly rash (acrodermatitis enteropathica), diarrhea, hair loss, altered taste perception, poor wound healing, impaired immune competence, eye lesions

1.4.6   Ultra-trace elements

(No proven essentiality in humans)

Aluminum	Modulates enzymes in Krebs cycle and glutamate dehydrogenase; contaminant in manufactured solutions with toxic tissue accumulation
Arsenic	Methylation of biomolecules (eg, histones), conversion of methionine to taurine and polyamines; toxicity related to swapping for phosphate in enzyme reactions: uncouples oxidative phosphorylation and causes DNA instability; fish grain, cereals
Boron	Bone and mineral metabolism; found in non-citrus fruits, leafy green vegetables, pulses
Bromine	Incorporated into peroxidases (eg, vanadium haloperoxidase); kelp, seaweed, nut, some baked goods
Cadmium	Transcriptional regulator, cell signaling; toxicity related to reactive oxygen species
Cobalt	No additional requirement above B12 requirements; toxicity related to inhibition of mitochondrial dehydrogenase and cardiomyopathy
Fluorine	Dental and skeletal health; G-protein activator; aluminum- and beryllium-fluoride complexes are phosphate analogs
Germanium	Thought to be an antioxidant; toxicity related to renal failure; garlic mushrooms, onions, bran, vegetables, seeds, meats, dairy
Lithium	Affects various enzymes (eg, tyrosine and tryptophan hydroxylases) and hormones (vasopressin, aldosterone, thyroid, parathyroid); grains and vegetables
Nickel	Enzyme cofactor in proprionate pathway of branched-chain amino acid and odd-chain fatty acid metabolism; chocolate, nuts, dried beans, peas, and grains
Rubidium	Can act as replacement for potassium; fruits and vegetables
Silicon	Cartilage calcification, crosslinking macromolecules (eg, osteonectin); whole high fiber grains, cereals, root vegetables
Tin	Redox reactions, protein complexes; fruits and vegetables
Vanadium	Participates in receptor phosphorylation (eg, insulin receptor); shellfish, mushrooms, black pepper, dill seed

1.4.7 Dietary reference intakes

For Vitamins & Minerals in Adults*
See also Dietary Reference Intakes (DRIs) →246

Nutrient (mg)	RDA	AI	TUL
A	0.700 - 1.300	-	2.800-3.000
D	-	0.005-0.015	0.100
E	15-19	-	800-1000
K	-	0.075-0.120	ND
B1	1.0-1.4	-	ND
B2	1.0-1.6	-	ND
B3	14-18	-	30-35
B5	-	5-7	ND
B6	1.2-2.0	-	80-100
B7	-	0.025-0.035	ND
B9	0.400-0.600	-	0.800-1.000
B12	0.0024-0.0028	-	ND
C	65-120	-	1800-2000
Choline	-	400-550	3000-3500
Ca	-	1000-1300	2500-3000
Cl	-	1800-2300	3400-3600
K	-	4700-5100	ND
Mg	310-420	-	350**
Na	-	1200-1500	2300
Phos	700-1250	-	3000-4000
Cu	0.890-1.300	-	8-10
Cr	-	0.020-0.045	ND
Fe	8-27	-	40-45
I	0.150-0.290	-	0.9-1.1
Mb	0.043-0.050	-	1.7-2.0
Mn	-	1.6-2.6	9-11
Se	0.055-0.070	-	0.150-0.400
Zn	8-14	-	34-40

Nutrient (mg)	RDA	AI	TUL
As	-	ND	ND
Al	-	ND	ND
Bo	-	ND	17-20
Br	-	ND	ND
Cd	-	ND	ND
Co	-	ND	ND
F	-	ND	ND
Ge	-	ND	ND
Li	-	ND	ND
Ni	-	ND	0.6-1.0
Rb	-	ND	ND
Si	-	ND	ND
Sn	-	ND	ND
Va	-	ND	1800

* Normal ranges inclusive for adults (young to old), men and women, pregnancy, and lactation; ND - not determinable (from Institute of Medicine; www.iom.edu)
** TUL from a Mg supplement only (not including dietary Mg)
AI - adequate intake; TUL - tolerable upper intake level

1.5   Dietary Supplements

1.5.1   Definition[6]

Dietary supplements (DS) include vitamins and mineral, herbs and other phyto-chemicals, amino acids, dietary substances that supplement the diet by increas-ing the total dietary intake (eg, enzymes, organ tissue, glandulars), concentrates, metabolites, concentrates or extracts; dietary supplements may generally be ob-tained without a prescription

1994 Dietary Supplement Health and Education Act (DSHEA)

- Manufacturers do not need to register their products with the FDA nor get FDA approval before producing or selling dietary supplements.
- Manufacturers must make sure that product label information is "not false and misleading."
- Purpose of DSHEA:
  - Allow customers access to safe dietary supplements
  - Improve the health of Americans
  - Empower customers to make choices about preventative health
  - Stimulate growth of the industry

2006 Dietary supplement and nonprescription drug consumer protection act

Mandates reporting serious adverse events associated with use of the product

2007 Current good manufacturing practices for the supplement industry

Manufacturers must have proper controls in place so that supplements are processed in a consistent manner, and meet quality standards as to identity, purity, strength, and composition

FDA may issue adverse event reports/warnings related to DS

Types of claims allowed on DS labels

- Nutrient-content (eg, "high in calcium")
- Structure-function or nutrition support (eg, "calcium builds bone")
- Disease claim (eg, "decreases risk of osteoporosis") - however, this requires FDA authorization based on review of scientific evidence; examples:
  - Calcium: ↓ risk of osteoporosis
  - Fiber: ↓ risk of cancer
  - Folic acid: ↓ risk of neural tube defects
  - Soy protein: ↓ risk of coronary heart disease

56   1 Diet, Food & Supplements

Nutraceuticals

- DS containing concentrated form of a bioactive substance originating from a food, but packaged in a non-food matrix
- Used to enhance health in doses greater than those found in normal foods
- Example: DS (soy protein) versus Nutraceutical (ipriflavone)

Problems with DS

- Patients fail to report use to their physicians
- Adverse interactions with medications and other DS, for example:
  - Insulin and chromium
  - Spironolactone and licorice
  - Warfarin and ginkgo biloba
- Intrinsic risks unknown due to insufficient scientific substantiation
- Mislabeling:
  - Omission of adulterating substances that are harmful or interfere with the absorption or action of the active substance
  - Inclusion of active substances not present
  - Misrepresentation of quantities of active substances
  - Unsubstantiated disease claim

General recommendation

DS should only be considered when net proven benefit is greater than expected risk

1.5.2   Summary of common DS

Alpha-lipoic acid (ALA)	Proven benefit in diabetic neuropathy
Carnitine	Dipeptide (lysine + methionine) useful in carnitine depleted states (hepato-renal insufficiency, parenteral nutrition, valproate)
Choline	Required nutrient and ↑ intake recommended for pregnant women to support fetal brain development
Chromium	Interacts with chromodulin and can ↑ insulin action; no proven net benefit in patients with diabetes
Coenzyme Q10	Functions in electron transport; proven benefits for statin-induced myopathy, mitochondrial disorders, congestive heart failure, and ischemia-reperfusion injury

Summary of common DS (cont.)	
Creatine	May be useful in McArdle's disease (glycogen storage disease type V)
Dehydro-epiandrosterone (DHEA) & androstenedione	Insufficient evidence to manage disease states
Fish oil and omega-3 fatty acids	Proven benefit for hypertriglyceridemia
Flavonoids isoflavones, and ipriflavone	Phenolic compounds in plants; insufficient evidence to treat disease states, but the benefits of soy protein as part of a healthy diet are well documented
Glucosamine and chondroitin	Weak evidence demonstrating benefit for osteoarthritis
Glutamine	Conditionally essential/indispensible amino acid with some studies demonstrating benefits in critical illness
Kelp	No benefit for treatment of thyroid disease
Melatonin	Indoleamine with some studies demonstrating efficacy in improving sleep
Phytosterols	Structure similar to cholesterol; proven benefits in hypercholesterolemia and secondary prevention after an atherosclerotic event
Probiotics	Specific products have proven benefits in inflammatory bowel disease, infectious colitis, pouchitis, irritable bowel syndrome
Saw palmetto (Serenoa repens berry extract)	Insufficient evidence as first-line therapy for benign prostatic hypertrophy
Selenium	Limited evidence of benefit of 100 mcg BID in Graves orbitopathy; possible benefit for prevention of postpartum thyroid dysfunction
Taurine	Conditionally essential/indispensible amino acid with inconclusive benefits for parenteral nutrition related hepatopathy
Tyrosine	Unproven thyromimetic effects

1.5.3   Protein supplements

Glutasolve powder

Manufacturer	Nestle
Ingredients	L-glutamine, Maltodextrin
Serving/packet	15 g/packet
Uses	• Nutrition support of patients with malabsorption • GI disorders associated with GI Surgery, chemotherapy and radiation, inflammatory bowel disease, HIV/AIDS, infectious enteritis, impaired immune function or metabolic stress states, severe burn injuries, trauma, post-op recovery
Appropriate for these diets	Lactose free, gluten free, Kosher

Arginaid powder

Manufacturer	Nestle
Serving/packet	4.5 g l-arginine and vitamin C 156 mg and vitamin E 90 IU/packet 25 kcal
Uses	Nutrition support of patients with pressure ulcers, diabetic foot ulcers, venous ulcers, burn injuries, non-healing surgical wounds
Flavors	Cherry and orange flavors
Appropriate for these diets	Lactose free, gluten free, Kosher

Beneprotein

Manufacturer	Nestle
Ingredients	Whey Protein Isolate (milk), Soy Lecithin
Nutritional information	100% whey protein (milk protein)
Serving/packet	Contains 6 g/serving (1 scoop)
Appropriate for these diets	Lactose free, gluten free
Preparation	Can mix into food and beverages or flush through feeding tube in 2-4 oz water

Juven	
Manufacturer	Abbott
Dosage	2 packets per day
Flavor	Unflavored, fruit punch, orange
Serving/packet	7 g 1-arginine, 7 g l-glutamine, 4 g carbohydrate
Uses	Nutrition support of patients recovering from surgery or with wounds
Appropriate for these diets	Lactose free
Preparation	Can add to 8 oz water or juice or add to apple sauce or ice cream or in mix in 4 oz water to administer through feeding tube

Promod	
Manufacturer	Abbott
Flavor	Ready to drink fruit punch flavor
Type	Liquid protein- hydrolyzed collagen
Serving/packet	100 kcal and 10 g protein per oz

1.5.4 Probiotics

Florastor	
Manufacturer	Biocodex Inc.
Type	Probiotic: single strain Saccharomyces boulardii (yeast probiotic). Available as capsule or packet
Dosage	One capsule twice a day
Uses	Antibiotic associated diarrhea, acute infectious diarrhea
Contraindicated	In patients with a central line
Refrigeration	Does not require
Prescription	Does not require

VSL#3

Manufacturer	Sigma Tau
Type	Probiotic mixture High potency probiotic medical food
Dosage	IBS: 2-4 capsules/day or 1 packet per day UC: 4-8 capsules per day or 1-2 packets per day, 1 DS packet Active UC: 2-4 packets or 1-2 DS packets Ileal pouch (pouchitis): 2-4 packets per day or 1-2 DS
Uses	Dietary management of ileal pouch, ulcerative colitis and irritable bowel
Appropriate for these diets	Vegetarian, gluten free, kosher, halal, dairy free
Prescription	Requires
Store	Should be refrigerated; can be left at room temperature for up to 2 weeks

1.5.5   Other

MCT oil

Manufacturer	Nestle
Source	Modified coconut and palm kernel oil
Nutritional information	1t bsp (15 ml) has 115 kcal, 14 g fat
Dosage	Maximum 100 mL/day, maximum 20 mL/dose
Uses	Fat calories for patients with chyle leak Can mix in juice or milk use in sauces or salad dressing
Appropriate for these diets	Lactose free, gluten free, Kosher

Benefiber

Manufacturer	Novartis
Ingredients	Wheat dextrin soluble fiber (Gluten free)
Dosage	3 g fiber/4 oz serving
Other information	Can mix into hot or cold beverages (except carbonated) or cook with food

Levocarnitine (L-carnitor)	
Manufacturer	Sigma-Tau
Dosages	Supplied as 1g/5 ml single dose vial for iv administration, 330 mg tablets, 1g/10 ml oral solution • Metabolic disorder: 50 mg/kg slow iv bolus • ESRD: 10-20 mg/kg slow iv bolus after dialysis • Usual oral tablet dosage: 990 mg bid-tid • Usual oral solution dosage: 1-3 g (10-30 mL)/day in divided doses
Uses	Carnitine deficiency

1.6   Sports Nutrition

(see reference [7,8,9,10,11])

1.6.1   Hydration

Risks of dehydration and over-hydration

- Greater than 2% loss of total body weight with exercise impairs the cardiovascular (CV) response
- Intact CV response allows tissue perfusion and evaporative cooling via sweating
- Fluid replacement (commensurate with sweat losses) reduces risks of heat-related disorders and improves exercise performance
- Over-hydration with hypo-osmolar fluids leads to hyponatremia and potentially death:
  - Salt losses occur with sweating
  - ↑ risk with NSAIDs (acetaminophen is acceptable)

Prevention/treatment strategies for dehydration and salt loss

- Rehydration needs based on pre- and post-exercise weights is preferred
- Daily water requirements (based on 70 kg adult) is about 2 liters plus exercise related losses
- Pre-exercise hydration is often recommended with 1-2 (8 oz) glasses of water 2 hours before and ½-1 glass immediately prior to exercise if dark urine
- Fluid intake during exercise must be individualized
- 1-1.5 liters water required for every kg water lost after exercise
- Consume salty foods: pretzels, crackers; or salt tabs
- Marathon runners need 400-800 mg Na per hour with warm/hot weather

Emergency treatment of dehydration

Signs and symptoms:

- >2% water loss: thirst, fatigue, ↓ performance (up to 50%), cramping, decreased perspiration, flushing, hypotension, orthostasis, tachycardia, ↑ temperature (from decreased sweating)
- 5%-6% water loss: nausea, headache, somnolence
- 10%-15% water loss: spasticity, skin shriveling/wrinkling, vision dimming, urination reduced/painful, delirium, loss of consciousness, seizure
- >15% usually fatal

Early intervention can prevent progression:

- Cool-off
- Rehydration:
  - for minor dehydration: sports drinks containing electrolytes and carbohydrate; may need to supplement with salt tablets
  - for severe dehydration; IV rehydration with electrolyte solution
  - Avoid food until water replaced (water required for digestion)

Emergency treatment of severe hyponatremia

- Cerebral edema and death may occur with Na <126 mmol/L
- Confused/obtunded hyponatremic athlete is generally "acute" and "hypervolemic"
- Intervention: (as needed) intubation, water restriction, furosemide, hypertonic saline

1.6.2   Nutrition

Basic recommendations

Recommendations may vary depending on the type of exercise or sport

- Achieve and maintain a healthy body weight
- Consume less saturated fat
  - Choose healthy sources of essential fatty acids (EFA): flaxseed, olive, soy, canola oils, pumpkin/sunflower seeds, walnuts, leafy vegetables, salmon, catfish
- Consume sufficient protein, including non-animal sources, to support the activity and performance level:
  - Partially hydrolyzed shakes, especially with whey protein, are popular
  - For endurance athlete 1.0-1.4 g/kg/day
  - For strength athletes 1.4-1.6 g/kg/day
- Relatively higher proportion of carbohydrates required before, during and after exercise to delay the onset of fatigue, and enhance exercise capacity and endurance:

- Insufficient evidence to support "train low" (low carbohydrate intake during training) strategies
- Starches and fiber (pasta, rice, breads, cereals, whole grains, pulses) used to replete glycogen
- Fructose is not effective at raising glycogen stores

Daily carbohydrate intake

Mild training or athletes with large body mass	3-5 g/kg/day
Moderate training for 60-90 min	5-7 g/kg/day
Intense training for 1-3 hours	7-12 g/kg/day
Extreme training for >4-5 hours	10-12 g/kg/day

- Pre-event "carb loading" (up to 3 days): usually 7-12 g/kg/day
- No benefit to "carb loading" for events less than 90 min
- Pre-event meal 1-4 hours prior 1-4 g/kg
- Carbohydrate intake during hour before exercise is controversial

During exercise	if <30 min	no carbohydrates
	if 30-75 min	mouth rinse
	if 1-2 hours	30 g/hours
	>2-3 hours	60 g/hours
	>2.5 hours	90 g/hours

Post-exercise: 1-1.2 g/kg; and repeat each hour until normal meal schedule resumed

Dietary supplements[9]

Dietary supplements with demonstrated performance enhancing effects and reasonable safety profile

Creatine	• Increases exercise performance by increasing ATP resynthesis • Usually given as loading dose for 5-7 days followed by maintenance dose • Usually cycled for efficacy • Avoid if renal or liver dysfunction or individual at risk for renal dysfunction (ie., diabetes)
Sodium bicarbonate	Increases hydrogen ion buffering capacity, thereby delaying fatigue and increasing exercise performance

Dietary supplements (cont.)	
Caffeine	• Increases time to exhaustion through central and peripheral mechanisms • Mobilizes fat stores and stimulates working muscles to use fat as a fuel, which delays depletion of muscle glycogen and allows for prolonged exercise • Usual dose 5 mg/kg 1-2 hours pre-competition (equal to 2-3 cups of coffee) • Note: urinary caffeine concentrations of more than 12 mcg per mL and 15 mcg/mL, respectively is prohibited but IOC and NCAA
Carbohydrate-electrolyte beverages (sports drinks)	• Enhance performance when used during activity • Must contain sodium to help avoid hyponatremia • Fluids help avoid dehydration • Provide energy to working muscle • Can cause GI upset if too high in carbohydrate (optimal 5%-7% carbohydrate) • Sports drinks are acidic and high in sodium and can erode tooth enamel: should rinse with water after use • Multiple transportable carbohydrates results in higher oxidation rates than single carbohydrate
Branched chain amino acids	• Effects in studies are variable • Does not acutely enhance performance • May help with muscle repair and synthesis • May reduce muscle soreness and hasten recovery • Long term supplementation may increase strength and endurance measures

Commonly used supplements without proven benefit

• Beta hydroxyl beta methyl butyrate
• Chromium (unless deficient)
• Iron (unless deficient)
• Arginine

Prohibited substances with dangerous adverse effects

• Anabolic steroids
• Ephedrine
• Human growth hormone
• Erythropoietin

1.7   Food Allergies

1.7.1   General

- Immune reaction against a food protein
- More common in children (6%-8% of children age < 3 years), compared with adults (3%-4% of adults)
- Children typically outgrow food allergies over time:
  - 40% of children with atopic dermatitis have food allergies
  - Asthma and allergic rhinitis can worsen with certain foods
- Not a food intolerance (non-immune, usually due to a missing enzyme):
  - Lactose intolerance affects 1:10 people
  - Normal: not having lactase (being lactose intolerant)
  - Mutation: dominant inheritance to have lactase and tolerate milk (protective)
- Prevalence of particular food allergy in a country depends on prevalence of that particular food preference in that population
- Heat (cooking) increases the allergic potential
- Infants with severe milk allergy on formula can used hydrolyzed protein or free amino acid based formulas
- Some latex allergies cross-react with banana, kiwi, avocado, and other foods
- Food-associated exercise-induced anaphylaxis in adult female athletes <30 years old
  - Usually 2-4 hours after eating wheat or shellfish
  - Allergy only occurs with exercise

1.7.2   Common food allergens

- Cow's milk (some cross-reactivity with beef and/or soy; preschool age)
- Egg (white > yolk; preschool age and usually resolves by adulthood)
- Seeds (sesame, poppy, pumpkin, almond; protein in the oils; childhood)
- Peanuts (a bean; age 5-18 years)
- Fish, shellfish (adults)
- Tree nuts (adults)

1.7.3 IgE-mediated food allergy

- 90% of all food allergies
- Type-1 immediate hypersensitivity reaction
  - Certain proteins resist degradation in the GI tract
  - Some of these intact proteins elicit response of TH2 lymphocytes to produce interleukin-4 (IL-4)
  - The TH2 cells and IL-4 interact with B cells to produce IgE
  - IgE binds to Fc receptors (Fc RI) on mast cells and basophils (sensitization)
  - With further exposure, the allergen complexes with the IgE and activates the sensitized cells to degranulate and release histamine, prostaglandins, etc.
  - This causes the signs and symptoms of inflammation and the allergic response (local or systemic [anaphylaxis]; acute response)
  - Late phase responses occur 2-24 hours later
- Present with urticaria, angioedema, sweating, flushing, tearing, sneezing, coughing, nasal congestion, dizziness, nausea/vomiting, diarrhea, abdominal cramping/bloating, and/or anaphylaxis
- Oral (pollen-food) allergy syndrome
  - Reaction to fresh fruits, nuts, and/or vegetables (no reaction if cooked)
  - Most common food allergy
  - Cross-reactivity between the food and tree or weed pollen
- Ragweed with banana, melons, cucumber, zucchini
- Alder/birch pollen with almonds, hazelnuts, apples, cherries, strawberry, raspberry
- Signs limited to mouth, lips, tongue, and throat

1.7.4 Non-IgE-mediated food allergy

- Less severe and more delayed than IgE-mediated
- Primarily in intestinal mucosa with GI symptoms
  - Food protein-induced enterocolitis syndrome (FPIES)
  - Food protein proctocolitis/proctitis
  - Food protein-induced enteropathy (eg, celiac disease [response to gluten])
  - Milk-soy protein intolerance (MSPI; response to milk/soy protein during infancy)
  - Heiner syndrome: lung involvement (bleeding/hemosiderosis) after milk precipitins (milk protein - IgG complexes) enter circulation from GI

1.7.5 Mixed type

IgE-mediated and non-IgE-mediated

1.7.6   Diagnosis

- History
- Food challenges
- Trial of an "elimination" diet
  - 2 weeks for response if IgE-mediated
  - Up to 3 months for response if non-IgE-mediated
- Prick/puncture skin testing
- RAST (radioallergosorbent) test
- Differential: food intolerance (eg, lactose), celiac disease, irritable bowel syndrome, C1 esterase inhibitor deficiency

1.7.7   Treatment/management

- Avoid culprit
- Immunotherapy
- Anti-IgE therapy (omalizumab)
- Oral immunotherapy or tolerance induction
- Antihistamines, steroids, epinephrine autoinjector pen
- Need medical alert bracelet

1.8   Food Safety

(see reference [12])

1.8.1   General rules

- Use separate cutting boards and plates for produce and raw meat, poultry, seafood or eggs
- Separate raw meat, poultry, seafood, and eggs from other foods in your shopping cart and in the refrigerator to avoid contamination from dripping
- Refrigerate perishable foods and leftovers within 2 hours
- Keep refrigerator between 32-40 °F
- Keep freezer below 0 °F
- Always marinate in the refrigerator
- Do not thaw at room temperature (use refrigerator, cold water, microwave)

1.8.2 Cooking temperatures

Food category	Temperatures (use food thermometer)
Ground meat	160 °F
Ground poultry	165 °F
Fresh beef, veal, lamb	145 °F (rest 3 min)
Poultry	165 °F
Pork	145 °F (rest 3 min)
Fish	cook until opaque or 145 °F
Shellfish	cook until shells open (do not eat if shell does not open)
Eggs	cook until yolks and whites are firm (in recipes heat to 160 °F)

1.8.3 Storage

Food category	Temperatures
Eggs	3-5 weeks, do not freeze
Hard cooked eggs	1 week
Salads (ie, tuna, egg, chicken, macaroni, ham)	Refrigerate 3-5 days, do not freeze
Hot dogs	Refrigerate 1 week, freeze 1-2 months
Luncheon meat	Refrigerate 3-5 days, freeze 1-2 months
Bacon	Refrigerate 7 days, freeze 1 month
Sausage	Refrigerate 1-2 days, freeze 1-2 months
Ground meat	Refrigerate 1-2 days, freeze 3-4 months
Steaks	Refrigerate 3-5 days, freeze 6-12 months
Chicken	Refrigerate 1-2 days, freeze 9 months
Seafood	Refrigerate 1-2 days, freeze 2-3 months if fatty, 6-8 months if lean
Leftovers	refrigerate 3-4 days, cooked meat freeze 2-6 months, chicken nuggets freeze 1-3 months, pizza freeze 1-2 months

1.8.4   Shopping hints

- Make sure canned goods are free of dents, cracks, or bulging lids
- Purchase produce that is not bruised
- Check the "sell by" or "use-by" dates on perishable foods
- Choose pasteurized dairy and refrigerated juice products

1.8.5   Washing rules

- Wash surfaces and utensils in hot soapy water after each use
- Can use 1 tablespoon unscented chlorine bleach in 1 gallon of water to sanitize
- Wash hands with soap after handling food
- Wash fruits and vegetables in water including the skin even if you plan to peel
- Do not wash meat, poultry or eggs before cooking

List of references

1. Dietary Guidelines for Americans 2010 U.S. Department of Agriculture?U.S. Department of Health and Human Services www.dietaryguidelines.gov
2. Mechanick JI, Brett EM (eds) January 2010 Power of Prevention: The Complete Guide to Lifelong Nutrition. Amazon.com
3. Therapeutic Lifestyle Changes. 2005 National Institutes of Health Publication. www.nhlbi.nih.gov/health/public/heart/chol/chol_tlc.pdf
4. Pecoits-Filho R, Lindholm B, Stenvinkel P: The malnutrition, inflammation and atherosclerosis (MIA) syndrome- the heart of the matter. Nephrol Dial Transplant 2002;17(suppl11)28-31.
5. National Research Council. Weight Gain During Pregnancy: Reexamining the Guidelines. Washington, DC: The National Academies Press, 2009.
6. Mechanick et al. Endocrine Pract 2003; 9: 417-470.
7. Smith EL, Mechanick JI. Hydration and nutrition for the athlete. In, Herrera JE, Cooper G (eds.) Essention Sports Medicine. Humana Press, Totowa NJ, 2008, pp. 175-186
8. Jeukendrup, AE Nutrition for endurance sports: Marathon, triathlon, and road cycling Journal of Sports Sciences, 2011; 29(S1): S91-S9
9. Jenkinson DM, Harbert AJ Supplements and sports. Am Fam Physician. 2008 Nov 1;78(9):1039-46.
10. Heneghan C, Gill P, O'Neill B, Lasserson D, Thake M, Thompson M.Mythbusting sports and exercise products. BMJ 2012;345:e4848
11. Burke LM: Fueling strategies to optimize performance: training high or training low? Scand J Med Sci Sports 2010: 20 (Suppl. 2): 48-58
12. http://www.foodsafety.gov/

2   Differential Diagnosis

2.1   Obesity

Definition:
Obesity is a disease with characteristic signs, symptoms, and morbidities
including increase in body fat (associated with abnormal body composition), and
abnormally high adipose tissue (subcutaneous, visceral, ectopic). Obesity is
gauged by the body mass index (BMI), which is equal to weight/height^2 in kg/m^2.

BMI (kg/m^2)	
Normal	18.5–24.9
Overweight	25–29.9
Obesity Class I	30–34.9
Obesity Class II	35–39.9
Obesity Class III	≥40

Waist circumference (WC) and WHR cutoffs (for Asians*)				
	BMI (kg/m^2)	Obesity class	WC: M ≤90 cm F ≤80 cm	WC: M >90 cm F >80 cm
Underweight	<18.5	–	–	–
Normal	18.5–22.9	–	Average	Average
Overweight	23–24.9	I	Increased	High
Obesity	25.0–29.9	II	High	Very high
			Very high	Very high
Extremely Obese	≥30	III	Severe	Severe
Waist to hip ratio				
Male	≥0.9			
Female	≥0.8			

* China, Southeast Asia, and India
Jeffrey I. Mechanick, Curr Diab Rep. Diabetes-Specific Nutrition Algorithm: A Transcultural
Program to Optimize Diabetes and Prediabetes Care 12(2): 180–194 copyright © 2012 April.

A high body mass index is associated with increased risk of death at all ages among both men and women.
See also weight gain →73

Contributory factors	• Familial influences
	• Physical inactivity
	• Dietary factors:
	  – Eating patterns
	  – Type of diet
	• Socioeconomic
	• Educational:
	  – Maternal nutritional factors
	  – Infant feeding practices
	• Cultural-ethnic
	• Psychologic
	• Sleep deprivation

Genetic factors	• Inherited predisposition
	• Congenital leptin deficiency (very rare)
	• POMC deficiency (very rare)- present with adrenal crisis, pale skin
	• Melanocortin 4 receptor mutation- may account for up to to 6% of nonsyndromic severe early onset obesity, associated with increased height, insulin resistance, increased bone mineral density
	• Epigenetic
	• Genetic syndromes associated with obesity:
	  – Alström's syndrome (retinal dystrophy, deafness, DM)
	  – Dystrophia adiposogenitalis (Fröhlich's syndrome) (hypogonadotropic hypogonadism, hypothalamic obesity)
	  – Bardet-Biedl syndrome (mental retardation, dysmorphic extremities, retinal dystrophy or retinitis pigmentosa, hypogonadism)
	  – Prader-Willi syndrome (microsomia, obesity, imbecility, muscular hypotension, bilateral cryptorchidism, hypogonadotropic hypogonadism)
	  – MEHMO (X-linked mitochondrial inheritance, mental retardation, epilepsy, hypogenitalism, microcephaly, obesity
	  – Cohen syndrome (microcephaly, hypotonia, retinal dystrophy)

Genetic factors (cont.)	– Wilson-Turner (mental retardation, gynecomastia) – Stewart-Morel-Morgagni syndrome (hyperostosis frontalis interna, hirsutism, virilism, menstrual irregularities, DM)
Hypothalamic dysfunction	• Tumor • Inflammation • Trauma • Surgery • Increased intracranial pressure

Endocrine	• Hypothyroidism
	• Cushing's syndrome
	• Hyperinsulinism:
	  – Insulinoma
	  – Excess exogenous insulin
	• Hypogonadism: (reduced estrogen may contribute to central adiposity in men and women)
	• Polycystic ovary syndrome (hirsutism, menstrual abnormalities, infertility, enlarged "polycystic ovaries")
	• Pubertal obesity

Lipomatosis	Excessive local accumulation of fat: • Multiple lipomas • Madelung's disease • Launois-Bensaude syndrome • Adiposis dolorosa (Anders' disease, Dercum's disease)

Drugs	• Psychiatric or neurologic agents:
	  – Antipsychotic agents: Phenothiazines, olanzapine, clozapine, risperidone
	  – Mood stabilizers lithium
	  – Antidepressants: Tricyclics, MAOIs, some SSRIs, mirtazapine
	  – Antiepileptic drugs: Gabapentin, valproate, carbamazepine
	• Steroid hormones: Corticosteroids, Progestational steroids
	• Antidiabetes agents: Insulin, sulfonylureas, thiazolidinediones

Drugs (cont.)	• Antihypertensive agents: β_1-Adrenergic and α_1-adrenergic receptor blockers • Antihistamines: cyproheptadine • HIV Protease inhibitors
Miscellaneous	• Glycogen storage disorders • Pregnancy

2.2   Weight Gain

See also obesity →70

Causes	

• Sedentary lifestyle
• Fluid overload
• Discontinuation of smoking
• Endocrine, metabolic:
  – Hypothyroidism
  – Hyperinsulinism
  – Maturity-onset diabetes mellitus
  – Cushing's syndrome
  – Hypogonadism
  – Hypothalamic disorder
	• Drugs:
	  – Glucocorticoids
	  – Nutritional supplements
	• Anxiety disorder with compulsive eating
	• Binge eating disorder
	• Bulimia
	• Congenital diseases

2.3   Weight Loss

See also anorexia →74

Insufficient nutrition	• Malnutrition
	• Malassimilation:
	  – Maldigestion
	  – Malabsorption
	• Mechanical obstruction
	• Starvation
	• Loss of appetite:
	  – Carcinoma
		• Cardiac cachexia
		• Medications
		• Achalasia
		• Stenosis in the gastrointestinal tract
		• Chronic diseases:
		• Hepatopathy; Renal failure

Reduced absorption	• Malabsorption • Chronic diarrhea	• Proximal fistula • Celiac sprue

Losses	• Intestinal parasites: – Vomiting • Bacterial overgrowth • Intestinal fistula	• Hyperemesis gravidarum • Poorly controlled diabetes mellitus
Increased demand	• Critical illness, • Cachexia • Drugs	• Hyperthyroidism • Malignancy • Parasitic infection
Psychological	• Anorexia nervosa • Avoidant restrictive food intake disorder	• Rumination syndrome • Depression • Drugs/alcohol abuse
Infectious	• Tuberculosis	• HIV
Gastrointestinal	• Hepatobiliary diseases • Malassimilation • Achalasia • Pancreatitis • Inflammatory bowel disease • Cirrhosis	• After small intestine resection • After gastrectomy • Gastric outlet obstruction • Carcinoid syndrome • Mesenteric ischemia
Cardiovascular	• Heart failure: – Cardiac cachexia	• Infectious endocarditis
Endocrine	• Hyperthyroidism • Addison's disease • Diabetes mellitus	• Hypopituitarism • Carcinoid syndrome
Drugs	• Chemotherapeutics • Drug abuse • Hyperthyroidism factitia	• Amphetamines • Digoxin
Systemic	• Cachexia: – Malignant tumors • Uremia	• Polyarteritis nodosa • Autoimmune diseases • Alcoholism

2.4   Anorexia

Diminished appetite, aversion to food.
Anorexia nervosa is a disorder characterized by deliberate weight loss, induced and/or sustained by the patient. The disorder occurs most commonly in adolescent girls and young women, but adolescent boys and young men may be affected more rarely, as may children approaching puberty and older women up to the menopause.

See also weight loss →73

Risk factors	• Perfectionist • Obsessive-compulsive personality	• Socially withdrawn • High achiever
DDx	• Weight loss • Bulimia • Affective disorder • Anxiety disorder	• Major depression • Schizophrenia • Diabulemia

2.5 Iron

The total iron content of the body is approx. 38 mg/kg in women and 50 mg/kg in men. The iron stores in the body are: erythrocytes: approx. 3000 mg; myoglobin: approx. 120 mg; cytochromes: approx. 3-8 mg; liver/spleen: approx. 300-800 mg. Daily turnover through synthesis and conversion of hemoglobin is 25 mg. Uptake occurs mainly through resorption in the small intestine. Only bivalent iron is resorbed intestinally; bound iron is trivalent. Considerable iron loss is possible through menstruation and pregnancy.

Reference range	
Women	7-25 µmol/L
Men	9-27 µmol/L

Decreased serum iron	
Insufficient dietary iron	• Malnutrition • Alcoholism • Vegetarian/vegan • Unbalanced nutrition
Increased requirements	• Pregnancy • Lactation • Infants or small children
Inadequate iron absorption	• Gastric and/or intestinal resection • Celiac sprue • Malabsorption/Maldigestion of siderous foods

Decreased serum iron (cont.)	
Hypo- and atransferrinemia	• Nephrotic syndrome • Cirrhosis • Exudative enteropathy • Congenital deficiency

Increased iron loss	• Chronic gastrointestinal blood loss
	• Blood donor
	• Hemodialysis
	• Menstrual bleeding:
	  – Occult bleeding
	  – Heavy menstrual bleeding
	• Massive hemoglobinuria

Iron metabolism disorder	• Chronic inflammations • Acute inflammations • Infections • Neoplasms • Myocardial infarction • Stress • Uremia

Increased serum iron

- Idiopathic hemochromatosis
- Secondary hemochromatosis
- Ineffective erythropoiesis with ↑ destruction of red blood cells in the bone marrow
- Vitamin B12 deficiency
- Hemolysis
- Hemolytic anemia
- Hemosiderosis
- Sideroblastic anemia

- Homozygous thalassemia
- Megaloblastic anemia
- Porphyria cutanea tarda
- Frequent blood transfusions
- Nutritive iron overloading
- Hepatic hypersideremia in severe hepatopathy:
  – Release of stored iron through hepatocyte decay
- Cisplatin therapy

2.6   Folic Acid Deficiency

Deficiency of pteroylglutaminic acid
Part of the vitamin B complex, necessary for normal production of red blood cells.

Reference range	
Folic acid in serum/ plasma deficiency	3.6–15 mg/dL
Adequate folic acid supply	>4 mcg/L
Erythrocyte folic acid	120–800 mcg/L

Inadequate folate intake	• Alcohol abuse • Advanced age • Vegetarians • Malnutrition • Malabsorption	• Ulcerative colitis • Crohn's disease • Celiac disease • Postoperative (resection)

Increased Folate utilization	• Malignancy:
	  – Leukemias
	  – Solid tumors
	• Hyperthyroidism
	• Pregnancy
	• Lactation
	• Childhood
		• Psoriasis
		• ↑ erythropoiesis:
		  – Chronic blood loss
		  – Chronic hemolytic anemia
		  – Macrocytic anemia
		  – Other anemias

Miscellaneous	• Hematologic diseases • Enzyme defects	• Congenital impairment of folic acid metabolism
Drugs	• Alcohol • Chemotherapeutics • Contraceptives • Methotrexate • Pentamidine • Phenobarbitol • Phenytoin	• Primidone • Pyrimethamine • Sulfamethoxazole • Sulfasalazine • Triamterene • Trimethoprim

2.7 Calcium

Calcium (Ca) is required for the proper functioning of numerous intracellular and extracellular processes, including muscle contraction, nerve conduction, hormone release, and blood coagulation. In addition, calcium plays a unique role in intracellular signaling and is involved in the regulation of many enzymes.

Reference range	
Total calcium	8.5–10.4 mg/dL
Ionized calcium	1.1–1.4 mmol/L

The maintenance of Ca homeostasis, therefore, is critical. 55% of calcium is ionized in the plasma, 40% bound to protein, and 5% bound to organic acids. The concentration of ionized calcium, which represents the biologically active form, depends on the pH value and albumin concentration. Equation for estimation of ionized calcium:

Ionized calcium = measured calcium (mmol/L) 0.025 x albumin (g/L) + 1.0
Calcium + ((Normal Albumin - Serum Albumin) x 0.8)
Calcium / (0.6 + (Total Protein/8.5))

2.7.1 Hypercalcemia

An increase in total plasma calcium concentration above 10.4 mg/dL (2.60 mmol/L). Hypercalcemia usually results from excessive bone resorption. Regulation of serum concentration occurs through PTH, vitamin D and calcitonin. Symptoms in hypercalcemia include headaches, weakness, confusion, depression, hallucinations, psychosis, coma, hyporeflexia, bradycardia, shortened QT interval, hypertension, digitalis hypersensitivity with arrhythmias, nausea, vomiting, constipation, gastroduodenal ulcer disease, pancreatitis, insulin resistance, glucose intolerance, polyuria, polydipsia, nephrolithiasis, muscle weakness, chondrocalcinosis and vascular calcification.

Main causes	• Primary hyperparathyroidism
	• Tertiary hyperparathyroidism
	• Multiple myeloma
	• Humoral hypercalcemia of malignancy (elevated PTHrP)
	• Exogenous calcium and vitamin D
	• Sarcoidosis
	• Drugs

Increased uptake	• Milk-alkali syndrome • Vitamin D intoxication

Endocrine impairment	• Primary hyperparathyroidism (approx. 20%):
	  – Isolated or multinodal adenoma
	  – Parathyroid hyperplasia
	  – Carcinoma
	• Secondary/tertiary hyperparathyroidism:
	  – Acute and chronic kidney disease
	  – Autonomous hyperparathyroidism after long-term renal
	    failure. Parathyroid hyperplasia no longer controllable
	    due to calcemia
	• Hyperthyroidism
	• Cushing's syndrome
	• Adrenal failure
	• Acromegaly
	• Pheochromocytoma
	• VIPoma

Paraneoplastic syndrome (15%), secretion of osteolytic substances	• Tumors producing PTH:
	  – Ovarian cancer
	  – Bronchial carcinomas
	  – Kidney cancer
	• Interleukin-1, TNF alpha, osteoclast-activating factor in:
	  – Myeloma/lymphoma
	  – Secretion of prostaglandins

Osteolyses in malignant processes/bone infiltration/bone destruction (55%)	• Paget's disease with immobilization • Acute osteoporotic fracture with immobilization • Breast cancer • Multiple myeloma • Hodgkin's lymphoma • Leukemia • Polycythemia • Hepatocellular carcinoma

Drugs	• Aluminum intoxication • Lithium • Teriparatide • Theophylline • Thiazide diuretics • Vitamin A • Vitamin D (calcitriol) and Dihydrotachysterol [(A.T.10) which is a calcinosis factor] intoxication

Ectopic 1,25–dihydroxy–cholecalciferol production	• Granulomatous diseases
	  – Sarcoidosis
	  – Tuberculosis
	• Leprosy
	• Histoplasmosis
	• Coccidioidomycosis
	• Berylliosis
	• Oral candidiasis
	• Silicone-induced granuloma
	• Plasma cell granuloma

Reduced renal calcium excretion	• Familial hypocalciuric hypercalcemia • Thiazide diuretics • Dehydration
Miscellaneous	• Immobilization: – Paraplegia • Total parenteral nutrition • Acidosis

2.7.2 Hypocalcemia

Hypocalcemia is a decrease in total plasma calcium concentration below 8.5 mg/dL (2.12 mmol/L) in the presence of normal plasma protein concentration. Clinical signs of hypocalcemia include tetany, Chvostek's and Trousseau's signs, dystonia, aphasia, confusion, chorea-like motions, QT elongation, ↓ ST, heart failure, diarrhea, achlorhydria, malabsorption, muscle weakness, dry skin, hair loss and bilateral cataracts.

Main causes	• Hypoparathyroidism
	• Pseudohypoparathyroidism
	• Vitamin D deficiency
	• Renal failure
	• Magnesium depletion
	• Acute pancreatitis
	• Hypoproteinemia
	• Enhanced bone formation
	• Septic shock
	• Hyperphosphatemia
	• Drugs
Hypoalbuminemia	• Normal serum ionized calcium
Reduced uptake	• Malabsorption
	• Maldigestion
	• Short bowel syndrome
	• Vitamin D deficiency
Increased loss	• Alcohol abuse
	• Chronic renal failure
	• Nephrotic syndrome
	• Diuretic therapy
Endocrine	• Hypoparathyroidism
	• Congenital aplasia of the parathyroid gland
	• Idiopathic/autoimmune
	• Infiltrative
	• Postoperative after thyroidectomy
	• Pseudohypoparathyroidism
	• ↓ PTH effect on end organs/ endogenous resistance
	• Adrenocortical hyperplasia
	• Steroid therapy
Vitamin D deficiency (in secondary hyperparathyroidism)	• ↓ UV/sun
	• Malabsorption
	• Kidney diseases with reduced formation of activated vitamin D
	• Anticonvulsants

Hypomagnesemia	• Therapy with cisplatin • Therapy with aminoglycosides • Alcohol
Drugs	• Calcitonin • Cis platinum • Foscarnet, cinacalcet, bisphosphonates, denusomab • EDTA

Miscellaneous	• Sepsis
	• Alkalosis
	• Acute pancreatitis
	• Chronic renal failure
	• Nephrotic syndrome
	  – ↓ total calcium with normal ionized calcium
	• Hyperphosphatemia
	  – Phosphate administration: enemas, laxatives;
	    intravenous administration
	  – Renal failure
	  – Rhabdomyolysis
	  – Tumor lysis syndrome
	• Transfusion of citrated blood
	  – Osteoblastic metastases

2.8   Nutritional Anemias

Microcytic anemia	• Iron deficiency
	• Copper deficiency
	• Contribution of vitamin A and Vitamin E to iron
	  deficiency anemia
	• DDX: thalassemia trait, anemia of chronic disease/
	  inflammation, sideroblastic anemia

Macrocytic anemia	• vitamin B12 deficiency
	• folic acid deficiency
	• copper deficiency
	• DDX: alcoholism, liver diseases, hemolysis or bleeding,
	  hypothyroidism, exposure to chemotherapy drugs,
	  myelodysplasia

2.9   Skin Rash with Malnutrition

Essential fatty acid deficiency	Generalized and perioral dry thickened erythematous or pigmented desquamating plaques, generalized xerosis, dark brown plate like plaques • Necrolytic migratory erythema
Vitamin C deficiency (Scurvy)	Non-palpable non-thrombocytopenic purpuric rash and gingival hypertrophy • Coagulation disorders • Vasculitis • Cryoglobulinemia
Zinc deficiency	Well-demarcated, pustular and bullous or eczematous dermatitis in the perioral and acral regions • Seborrheic dermatitis • Necrolytic migratory erythema
Niacin deficiency	Photosensitive, pressure sensitive, erythematous, scaly and bullous skin rash involving the face, neck (Casal necklace), dorsal surface of the hands, and feet, fades with dusky brown-red coloration • Sunburn • Necrolytic migratory erythema • Carcinoid syndrome (tryptophan diverted to serotonin synthesis)

2.10   Hair Loss

Nutritional causes	• Essential fatty acid deficiency • Folate deficiency • Iron deficiency • Zinc deficiency • Vitamin D deficiency • Vitamin B12 deficiency: gray hair • Niacin B3 deficiency • Vitamin A toxicity • Selenium deficiency: hypopigmented hair • Copper deficiency: hypopigmented hair and pili torti • Vitamin C deficiency: corkscrew hair, perifollicular hyperkeratosis

Nutritional causes (cont.)	• Biotin deficiency (rare) • Low calorie diet/malabsorption • Low protein diet/malabsorption
Female pattern hair loss	(Gradual thinning on top of head with preservation of hair line) • Hyperandrogenism • Menopause • Withdrawal of oral contraceptives
Telogen effluvium (transient, diffuse, non-scarring)	• Acute illness • Post Surgery • Rapid weight loss • Thyroid dysfunction • Postpartum
Autoimmune (nonscarring)	• Systemic lupus erythematosus • Alopecia areata: patchy • Alopecia totalis
Scarring alopecia	• Frontal fibrosing • Lichen planopilaris • Discoid lupus • Other primary cicatricial alopecias
Drugs	Chemotherapies, interferon, lithium, valproic acid, fluoxetine, enoxaparin, beta blockers, ACE inhibitors, retinoids, isoniazide, etanercept, norgestrel, levonorgestrel

Phosphorus- as phosphate, it is a component of DNA, RNA, ATP and phospholipids that are components of cell membranes

2.11 Hyperphosphatemia

• Chronic kidney disease
• Phosphate containing laxatives
• Hypoparathyroidism
• Tumor lysis syndrome
• Familial tumoral calcinosis
• Fibroblast growth factor 23 deficiency
• Vitamin D toxicity
• Acromegaly
• Rhabdomyolysis
• Transfusion

2.12 Hypophosphatemia

- Hyperparathyroidism
- Refeeding syndrome
- Vitamin d deficiency
- Malnutrition
- X-linked hypophosphatemic rickets
- Fanconi's syndrome
- Hemodialysis
- Diarrhea
- Vomiting
- Phosphate binding antacids
- Alcohol abuse
- Diuretics
- Hungry bone syndrome
- Tumor produced Fibroblast growth factor 23

2.13 Congestive Heart Failure

Nutritional causes	• Selenium deficiency (Keshan's disease) • Thiamine deficiency (Beriberi) • Carnitine deficiency • Hypocalcemic rickets	• Copper deficiency • Zinc deficiency • Iron deficiency anemia • Hypokalemia • Hypomagnesemia • Cobalt toxicity
Other causes	• Idiopathic • CAD • HIV • Peripartum • Alcohol • Amyloidosis	• Connective tissue disease • Familial • Myocarditis • Drug induced

3   Malnutrition, Syndromes & Assessment

3.1   Nutritional Syndromes

3.1.1   Marasmus type of protein-energy malnutrition (PEM)

- Pure starvation with reduced food intake or assimilation; loss of body cell mass without an underlying inflammatory condition
- Weight loss usually >10% of usual weight
- Visceral proteins are preserved until severe starvation manifests
- Extracellular fluid is not increased
- Lean mass (fat-free mass [eg, muscle]; intracellular fluids) is decreased
- Fat mass is decreased
- Eg, anorexia nervosa
- Nutritionally responsive

3.1.2   Adult "Kwashiorkor-like" PEM

- Loss of body cell mass with inflammation
- Weight loss usually <10% of usual weight, or weight gain
- Visceral proteins are depleted
- Insulin resistance, futile substrate cycling with increased lipolysis and proteolysis
- Extracellular fluid is increased (third spacing) due to low plasma oncotic pressure
- Lean mass is decreased
- Fat mass is variably ↓ or preserved
- Eg, critical illness
- Only partially nutritionally responsive

3.1.3   Mixed marasmic-kwashiorkor PEM

- Semistarvation due to reduced energy and protein intake resulting from a systemic Inflammatory response
- Weight loss and hypoalbuminemia present
- Visceral proteins are reduced
- Extracellular fluid may be increased
- Lean mass is decreased
- Fat mass is usually decreased
- Only partially nutritionally responsive

3.1.4 Cachexia

Involuntary loss of body cell mass with an underlying persistent cytokine-mediated inflammatory disease or condition-similar to kwashiorkor-type PEM

3.1.5 Wasting

Involuntary loss of weight due to any cause

3.1.6 Sarcopenia

Involuntary loss of muscle mass, generally seen in geriatric patients

3.2 Physiology of Malnutrition

(see reference [13])

- Cytokines promote muscle catabolism, inhibit protein synthesis and muscle repair
- Anorexia induced by cytokines (eg, tumor-necrosis factor or "cachectin") accompanies inflammation and further promotes loss of lean tissue
- Acute phase metabolic response elevates REE
- Efficiency of dietary protein use is decreased
- Extracellular fluid compartment is expanded as oncotic pressure is lower with visceral protein depletion:
  – ↓ protein synthesis
  – ↑ vascular permeability
  – Albumin > globulin > fibrinogen are major determinants of plasma oncotic pressure
    – Albumin is reverse-phase reactant (anabolic)
    – Half-life is normally 20 days but serum levels can lower within 24 hours of injury due to rapid third spacing, ↑ metabolic clearance, and acute halting of gene expression - all under the influence of inflammatory cytokines
    – Non-nutrition factors have greater influence on albumin than dietary protein intake or overall nutritional status

3.3 Diagnosis of Malnutrition

(see reference [14])

- Insufficient energy intake to meet metabolic demands
- Unintentional weight loss
- Abnormal body composition:
  - Loss of muscle mass
  - Loss of subcutaneous fat
  - Generalized (anasarca) or localized fluid accumulation
- Diminished functional or performance status as measured by hand grip strength; "frailty"

Elements of History

• Dietary intake recall	• Disease state
• Weight loss	• Functional/performance status

Clinical Signs

• Fever	• Hair, skin, mouth, tongue
• Hypothermia	• Edema (can mask weight loss)
• Tachycardia	• Skin fold
• Muscle	• Arm circumference
• Subcutaneous Fat	• BIA, DXA, CT, MRI

Laboratory

• Albumin	• Leukocytosis
• Prealbumin	• Glucose
• CRP	• 24 hour UUN

Dietary Assessment

24 hour recall

Functional Outcome

• Grip strength	• Chair stand
• Gait	• Stair steps

3.4   Screening Tools

3.4.1   Subjective global assessment[15]

- Recommended by A.S.P.E.N.
- Based on:
  - Weight change: 2 weeks, 1 month, 6 months, 1 year
  - Dietary intake change
  - GI symptoms persisting daily over 2 weeks: Nausea, diarrhea, vomiting, dysphagia, anorexia
  - Functional impairment: Overall, duration, type
  - Physical exam: Muscle wasting (quadriceps, deltoid), subcutaneous fat loss (triceps, chest), edema (ankle, sacral, ascites)
  - Clinicians place patient into a category based on their subjective rating of the patient in history and physical examination
  - Score: Well nourished, mild/moderate undernutrition, severe undernutrition

3.4.2   Patient generated subjective global assessment[16]

- Designed for cancer patients
- Continuous scoring system
- Check-box format filled out by the patient plus physical exam
- Inquires about:
  - Weight change: 2 weeks, 6 months, 1 year
  - Symptoms of ↓ appetite, pain, nausea, diarrhea, vomiting, constipation, mouth sores, adverse smells, dry mouth, funny taste or no taste
  - Food intake
  - Activities and function
- Given numerical score plus a rating of well-nourished, moderately malnourished/suspected malnutrition, or severely malnourished
- Score ≥9 indicates need for urgent nutritional intervention[17]

3.4.3   Nutritional risk index[18]

- NRI= (1.519 x serum albumin g/dL) + (41.7 x present weight (kg)/usual body weight (kg)
- No risk >100
- Borderline malnourished (Mild risk) 97.5-100
- Mildly malnourished (Moderate risk) 83.5-97.5
- Severely malnourished (Major risk) <83.5

3.4.4 Nutrition risk score 2002[19]

- Recommended by E.S.P.E.N.
- Contains a grading of severity of disease as a reflection of increased nutritional requirements
- Includes four questions as a prescreening for departments with few at risk patients:
  - Performed only if lost of weight in past 3 months or BMI <20.5, reduced dietary intake or severely ill
- Includes age >70 as a risk factor
- Useful for all patients
- Numerical score based on:
  - Percent weight loss over 1-3 months
  - Food intake in preceding week
  - General condition
  - Current BMI
- Score of ≥3: Nutritionally at risk and nutrition care plan initiated
- Score of <3: Weekly rescreening of patient

3.4.5 Malnutrition screening tool[20]

- Developed for hospital use
- Simple
- High sensitivity and specificity
- Based on 3 main questions:
  - Have you been eating poorly because of ↓ appetite?
  - Have you lost weight recently without trying?
  - How much weight have you lost?
- Score of ≥2: at risk for malnutrition

3.4.6 Malnutrition universal screening tool (MUST)[21]

- Developed for use in the community but recently extended to hospital use
- Strong predictive validity for length of hospital stay, mortality in elderly wards and discharge destination in orthopedic patients
- Based on:
  - BMI
  - Weight loss in past 3-6 months
  - Presence of acute illness or anticipated NPO for 5 days
- 5 simple steps: Can be administered 3-5 min
- Patients categorized as low, medium or high risk based on numerical score

3.4.7 Mini Nutritional Assessment (MNA®)

Nestlé
Nutrition Institute

A	Has food intake declined over the past 3 months due to loss of appetite, digestive problems, chewing or swallowing difficulties?	Severe decrease in food intake	0
		Moderate decrease in food intake	1
		No decrease in food intake	2
B	Weight loss during the last 3 months	Weight loss greater than 3 kg (6.6 lbs)	0
		Does not know	1
		Weight loss between 1 and 3 kg (2.2 and 6.6 lbs)	2
		No weight loss	3
C	Mobility	Bed or chair bound	0
		Able to get out of bed/chair but does not go out	1
		Goes out	2
D	Has suffered psychological stress or acute disease in the past 3 months?	Yes	0
		No	2
E	Neuropsychological problems	Severe dementia or depression	0
		Mild dementia	1
		No psychological problems	2
F1	Body mass index (BMI): weight in kg/height in m^2	BMI less than 19	0
		BMI 19 to less than 21	1
		BMI 21 to less than 23	2
		BMI 23 or greater	3
If BMI is not available, replace question F1 with question F2. **Do not answer question F2 if question F1 is already completed.**			
F2	Calf circumference (CC) in cm	CC less than 31	0
		CC 31 or greater	3
		Score	

Screening score	
12–14	Normal nutritional status
8–11	At risk of malnutrition
0–7	Malnourished

References for Mini Nutritional Assessment (MNA):
i. Vellas B, Villars H, Abellan G, et al. Overview of the MNA® - Its History and Challenges. *J Nutr Health Aging.* 2006;10:456-465.
ii. Rubenstein LZ, Harker JO, Salva A, Guigoz Y, Vellas B. Screening for Undernutrition in Geriatric Practice: Developing the Short-Form Mini Nutritional Assessment (MNA-SF). *J. Geront.* 2001; 56A: M366-377
iii. Guigoz Y. The Mini-Nutritional Assessment (MNA®) Review of the Literature - What does it tell us? *J Nutr Health Aging.* 2006; 10:466-487.
iv. Kaiser MJ, Bauer JM, Ramsch C, et al. Validation of the Mini Nutritional Assessment Short-Form (MNA®-SF): A practical tool for identification of nutritional status. *J Nutr Health Aging.* 2009; 13:782-788.
® Société des Produits Nestlé, S.A., Vevey, Switzerland, Trademark Owners © Nestlé, 1994, Revision 2009. N67200 12/99 10M
For more information: www.mna-elderly.com

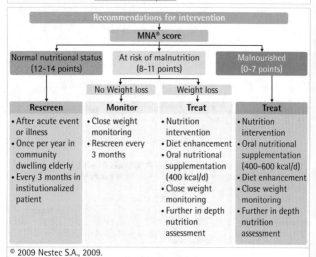

List of references

13 Jensen GL et al. Malnutrition syndromes: A Conundrum vs Continuum. JPEN 2009;33:710-716
14 White JV et al. Consensus statement: Academy of Nutrition and Dietetics and American Society for Parenteral and Enteral Nutrition: Characteristics Recommended for the identification and Documentation of Adult Malnutrition (undernutrition). JPEN 2012;36:275-283.
15 Detsky AS, McLaughlin JR, Baker JP, Johnston N, Whittaker S, Mendelson RA, Jeejeebhoy KN: What is subjective global assessment of nutritional status? 1987 JPEN;11:8-13, Copyright © 1987 by the American Society for Parenteral and Enteral Nutrition, Reprinted by Permission of SAGE Publications.
16 Ottery FS: Rethinking nutritional support of the cancer patient: the new field of nutritional oncology. Sem Oncol 21: 770-778.
17 Bauer J et al. use of the scored patient generated subjective global assessment as a nutrition assessment tool in patients with cancer. Eur J Clin Nutr 2002 56(8)779-785
18 The Veteran Affairs Total Parenteral Nutrition Cooperative Study Group. Perioperative Total parenteral nutrition in surgical patients. N Engl J Med; 1991:325:525-532.
19 Reprinted from J. Kondrup, S. P. Allison, M. Elia, B. Vellas, M. Plauth, ESPEN Guidelines for Nutrition Screening 2002, Clinical Nutrition, 22(4): 415-421, Copyright 2003, with permission from Elsevier.
20 Republished from Ferguson M, Capra S, Bauer J, Banks M: Development of a valid and reliable malnutrition screening tool for adult acute hospital patients, Nutrition, 15(6): 458-464, Copyright 1999, with permission from Elsevier.
21 Elia M Chairman and Editor (2003) Screening for malnutrition: A multidisciplinary responsibility: Development and Use of the "malnutrition Universal Screening Tool' 'MUST' for Adults. Malnutrition Advisory Group (MAG), a standing committee of BAPEN. Redditch, Worcs: BAPEN.

4   Overweight/Obesity

4.1   Obesity

4.1.1   Definitions

Body mass index

- Weight (kg)/height (m²)
- Weight (lbs)/height (in²) x 703

Classes of obesity

- Overweight BMI 25–29.9
- Obese class I BMI 30–34.9
- Obese class II BMI 35–39.9
- Obese class III BMI ≥40 (extreme/severe obesity)
- "Super obese" BMI ≥50
- BMI cutoffs are lower for Asians

Abdominal obesity

- Waist circumference >102 cm (40 in) men
- Waist circumference >88 cm (35 in) women
- Waist:hip ratio >0.8 in women
- Waist:hip ratio >0.9 in men
- Indians have more body fat for any given BMI compared with Caucasians and black Africans:
  - Waist >80 cm in women is risk for T2DM
  - Waist >90 cm in men is risk for T2DM

Pediatric ages 2–17

- Overweight: between 85–95 percentile
- Obese: above 95th percentile or BMI of 30 kg/m² or above

BMI

WEIGHT (left) × HEIGHT (top). Height shown as cm / inch.

kgs	lbs	147.3 4'10"	149.9 4'11"	152.4 5'0"	154.9 5'1"	157.4 5'2"	160 5'3"	162.5 5'4"	165.1 5'5"	167.6 5'6"	170.1 5'7"	172.7 5'8"	175.2 5'9"	177.8 5'10"	180.3 5'11"	182.8 6'0"	184.4 6'1"	187.9 6'2"
45.4	100	20.9	20.2	19.5	18.9	18.3	17.7	17.2	16.6	16.1	15.7	15.2						
47.6	105	22.0	21.2	20.5	19.8	19.2	18.6	18.0	17.5	17.0	16.5	16.0	15.5	15.1				
49.9	110	23.0	22.2	21.5	20.8	20.1	19.5	18.9	18.3	17.8	17.2	16.7	16.3	15.8	15.3			
52.2	115	24.0	23.2	22.5	21.7	21.1	20.4	19.8	19.1	18.6	18.0	17.5	17.0	16.5	16.0	15.6	15.3	
54.4	120	25.1	24.2	23.4	22.7	22.0	21.3	20.6	20.0	19.4	18.8	18.2	17.7	17.2	16.7	16.3	16.0	15.4
56.7	125	26.1	25.2	24.4	23.6	22.9	22.1	21.5	20.8	20.2	19.6	19.0	18.5	17.9	17.4	17.0	16.7	16.1
59.0	130	27.2	26.2	25.4	24.6	23.8	23.0	22.3	21.6	21.0	20.4	19.8	19.2	18.7	18.1	17.6	17.3	16.7
61.2	135	28.2	27.3	26.4	25.5	24.7	23.9	23.2	22.5	21.8	21.2	20.5	19.9	19.4	18.8	18.3	18.0	17.3
63.5	140	29.3	28.3	27.3	26.5	25.6	24.8	24.0	23.3	22.6	21.9	21.3	20.7	20.1	19.5	19.0	18.7	18.0
65.8	145	30.3	29.3	28.3	27.4	26.5	25.7	24.9	24.1	23.4	22.7	22.1	21.4	20.8	20.2	19.7	19.3	18.6
68.0	150	31.4	30.3	29.3	28.4	27.5	26.6	25.8	25.0	24.2	23.5	22.8	22.2	21.5	20.9	20.4	20.0	19.3
70.3	155	32.4	31.3	30.3	29.3	28.4	27.5	26.6	25.8	25.0	24.3	23.6	22.9	22.2	21.6	21.0	20.7	19.9
72.6	160	33.4	32.3	31.2	30.2	29.3	28.3	27.5	26.6	25.8	25.1	24.3	23.6	23.0	22.3	21.7	21.3	20.6
74.8	165	34.5	33.3	32.2	31.2	30.2	29.2	28.3	27.5	26.6	25.9	25.1	24.4	23.7	23.0	22.4	22.0	21.2
77.1	170	35.5	34.3	33.2	32.1	31.1	30.1	29.2	28.3	27.5	26.7	25.9	25.1	24.4	23.7	23.1	22.7	21.8
79.4	175	36.6	35.3	34.2	33.1	32.0	31.0	30.1	29.1	28.3	27.4	26.6	25.9	25.1	24.4	23.8	23.3	22.5
81.6	180	37.6	36.3	35.2	34.0	33.0	31.9	30.9	30.0	29.1	28.2	27.4	26.6	25.8	25.1	24.4	24.0	23.1
83.9	185	38.7	37.3	36.1	35.0	33.9	32.8	31.8	30.8	29.9	29.0	28.1	27.3	26.5	25.8	25.1	24.7	23.8
86.2	190	39.7	38.4	37.1	35.9	34.8	33.7	32.6	31.6	30.7	29.8	28.9	28.1	27.3	26.5	25.8	25.3	24.4
88.5	195	40.8	39.4	38.1	36.9	35.7	34.6	33.5	32.4	31.5	30.6	29.7	28.8	28.0	27.2	26.5	26.0	25.1
90.7	200	41.8	40.4	39.1	37.8	36.6	35.4	34.4	33.3	32.3	31.4	30.4	29.6	28.7	27.9	27.1	26.7	25.7
93.0	205	42.9	41.4	40.0	38.8	37.5	36.3	35.2	34.1	33.1	32.1	31.2	30.3	29.4	28.6	27.8	27.3	26.3
95.3	210	43.9	42.4	41.0	39.7	38.4	37.2	36.1	34.9	33.9	32.9	31.9	31.0	30.1	29.3	28.5	28.0	27.0
97.5	215	44.9	43.4	42.0	40.6	39.4	38.1	36.9	35.8	34.7	33.7	32.7	31.8	30.8	30.0	29.2	28.7	27.6
99.8	220		44.4	43.0	41.6	40.3	39.0	37.8	36.6	35.5	34.5	33.5	32.5	31.6	30.7	29.9	29.3	28.3
102.1	225		45.4	43.9	42.5	41.2	39.9	38.6	37.4	36.3	35.3	34.2	33.2	32.3	31.4	30.5	30.0	28.9
104.3	230			44.9	43.5	42.1	40.8	39.5	38.3	37.1	36.1	35.0	34.0	33.0	32.1	31.2	30.7	29.5
106.6	235			45.9	44.4	43.0	41.6	40.4	39.1	37.9	36.8	35.7	34.7	33.7	32.8	31.9	31.3	30.2
108.9	240				45.4	43.9	42.5	41.2	39.9	38.8	37.6	36.5	35.5	34.4	33.5	32.6	32.0	30.8
111.1	245					44.9	43.4	42.1	40.8	39.6	38.4	37.3	36.2	35.2	34.2	33.3	32.7	31.5
113.4	250					45.8	44.3	42.9	41.6	40.4	39.2	38.0	36.9	35.9	34.9	33.9	33.3	32.1

SI units:

$$BMI = \frac{mass\ (kg)}{(height\ (m))^2}$$

Imperial units:

$$BMI = \frac{mass\ (lb) \times 703}{(height\ (in))^2}$$

$$BMI = \frac{mass\ (lb) \times 4.88}{(height\ (ft))^2}$$

Legend: Underweight · Healthy · Overweight · Obese · Extremely obese

BMI of 13 kg/m² may indicate the turning point of the failure of the homeostasis mechanism in the starvation state and be the stage before the development of a serious physical crisis.

4.1.2   Pathophysiology

- Insulin and leptin circulate in levels in the bloodstream in proportion to body fat and interact with hypothalamic neurons in the arcuate nucleus of the hypothalamus
- Anabolic neurons when activated promote ↓ energy expenditure and ↑ food intake. These neurons coexpress neuropeptide Y (NPY) and agouti related peptide (AGRP) and are inhibited by leptin and insulin
- Catabolic neurons proopiomelanocortin (POMC) and cocaine and amphetamine related transcript (CART), release alpha MSH and when stimulated by leptin and insulin promote ↓ food intake. Alpha MSH binds to the melanocortin 4 receptor.
- Satiety signals are gut peptide secreted in response to the macronutrient content of an individual meal
    - CCK secreted from the duodenum
    - GLP-1 secreted by L cells of ileum and colon
    - Amylin secreted by pancreatic beta cells
    - Oxyntomodulin secreted by the L cells of distal ileum and colon
    - Peptide YY synthesized by L cells of distal ileum and colon
- Ghrelin is the only orexigenic gut hormone which is secreted from the stomach and duodenum and stimulates food intake
- New theories propose that an individual's gut microbiome and relative production of certain metabolites may predispose an individual to obesity[22]
- 2/3 of the US population is overweight or obese
- The incidence of overweight and obesity continues to rise worldwide with the highest prevalence in the US
- Obesity was recognized as a disease by the American Medical Association (AMA) for the first time in 2013
- Overweight and obesity increase the risk for many chronic diseases including: heart disease, stroke, hypertension, type-2 diabetes, osteoarthritis, as well as certain cancers including colon cancer, breast cancer and uterine cancer
- Related health care costs are estimated to reach over $800 billion by 2030

4.1.3   Weight loss goals

- 5%-10% body weight loss over 6-12 months
- 7% weight loss results is improvement in diabetes
- Early weight loss occurs due to diuresis (mechanism: lipolysis liberated water) in first 2 weeks

- Weight loss plateaus at 6 months: weight loss mechanisms occurs which take effect that oppose further loss[23]
  - Reduced spontaneous physical activity
  - ↑ metabolic efficiency
  - Reduced resting metabolic rate
  - ↑ skeletal work efficiency

4.1.4   Dietary modification

Low calorie meal plans

- 500-1000 kcal/day deficit results in 1-2 pounds weight loss per week
- Typically 800-1500 kcal/day

Very low calorie meal plans

- 600-800 kcal/day
- Requires physician supervision
- Should be limited to 12-16 weeks duration
- Requires high quality protein
- Requires micronutrient supplementation
- Contraindicated in pregnancy and lactation, major psychiatric disease, diabetes
- Consider prophylaxis for gallstone formation

Meal replacements

- Typically bars or shakes
- Replace 1-2 meals daily
- Calorie and portion controlled
- Fortified with vitamins and minerals
- Results in 2.5 kg more weight loss at 3 months than standard diet plan

4.1.5   Increased physical activity

- Can result in slightly increased weight loss of 4-5 kg by one year when coupled with dietary advice
- More important in the weight maintenance phase rather than in promotion of weight loss
- Reduces cardiometabolic risk
- 30 min exercise per day recommended
- 150 min moderate intensity activity or 75 min vigorous intensity activity per week recommended

4.1.6   Behavior therapy

- Self monitoring:
  - Portion controlled packaging
  - Read nutrition facts labels
  - Food and activity records
  - Can include data about feelings associated with eating
  - Helps detect disordered eating patterns
  - Revise unsuccessful regimens
  - Stay mindful
- Stimulus control:
  - Keep tempting foods out of sight
  - Limit eating to certain times, places
- Cognitive restructuring:
  - Learn to recognize and replace thoughts that combat weight loss efforts
  - Persevere despite failure days
- Group therapy:
  - Some patients respond well to support of others
  - Structure and responsibility of being at a meeting at a certain time
  - Others are also monitoring one's progress
  - Easy to implement (ie. join Weight Watchers, Jenny Craig)

4.1.7   Pharmacotherapy

Orlistat

See also drug chapter →215

Info	Mean weight loss 2.59 kg at 6 months and 2.89 kg at 12 months[24] Vitamin supplementation at night is recommended Fiber can reduce adverse effects

Phentermine

See also drug chapter →215

Info	Results in 5%-15% weight loss; can be used for up to 12 weeks; available since 1959

Lorcaserin

See also drug chapter →216

Info	Approved 2012; Efficacy: 47.2% and 42% lost 5% of body weight; 22.6% and 17.4% lost 10% of body weight; results in weight loss up to 8.1 kg[25]

Phentermine/topiramate	
See also drug chapter →216	
DO	3.75 mg/23 mg (phentermine 3.75 mg/topiramate 23 mg extended-release) daily for 14 days; then ↑ to 7.5 mg/46 mg daily Take once daily in the morning; avoid evening dose to prevent insomnia; discontinue or escalate if 3% weight loss is not achieved after 12 weeks on 7.5 mg/46 mg dose; discontinue if 5% weight loss is not achieved after 12 weeks on maximum daily dose of 15 mg/92 mg; discontinue 15 mg/92 mg dose gradually to prevent possible seizure; do not exceed 7.5 mg/46 mg dose for patients with moderate or severe renal impairment or patients with moderate hepatic impairment
Info	Approved 2012; at 56 weeks mean change in body weight was 8.1 kg with 7.5/46 mg and 10.2 kg with 15/92 mg[26]; mean percent change in weight after 108 weeks was 9.3% with 7.5/46 mg and 15/92 mg[27]

4.2   Bariatric Procedures

(see also obesity →94)

4.2.1   Role in comprehensive obesity management

Clinical practice guidelines

The following obesity and bariatric surgery clinical practice guidelines (CPG) describe a best practice and evidence-based role for bariatric surgery and serve as primary references for this section

2010 Scottish Intercollegiate Guidelines Network (SIGN)[28]

- Clinical assessment indicates high risk: patients with BMI >35 kg/m^2 or certain ethnic groups (eg, south Asians)
- Presence of ≥1 severe comorbidities that would have a meaningful clinical improvement with weight loss (eg, T2DM)
- Completion of a structured weight management program incorporating healthy eating, physical activity, behavioral therapy, and medications but not resulting in significant and sustained comorbidity improvement

2012 AACE/TOS/ASMBS[29]

- Patients with a BMI ≥40 kg/m^2, or ≥35 kg/m^2 with ≥1 severe comorbidity*, are eligible, provided bariatric surgery would not be associated with excessive risk
- Patients with BMI of 30-34.9 kg/m^2 with diabetes or metabolic syndrome may also be offered a bariatric procedure although current evidence is limited by the number of subjects studied and lack of long-term data demonstrating net benefit.

*Comorbidities: T2D, hypertension, hyperlipidemia, obstructive sleep apnea (OSA), obesity-hypoventilation syndrome (OHS), Pick-wickian syndrome (a combination of OSA and OHS), nonalcoholic fatty liver disease (NAFLD) or nonalcoholic steatohepatitis (NASH), pseudotumorcerebri, gastroesopha-geal refluxdisease (GERD), asthma, venous stasis disease, severe urinary incontinence, debilitating arthritis

Large studies demonstrating cardiovascular disease risk reduction and improvement in quality of life, surrogate markers

- Bariatric surgery candidates without diabetes or existing cardiovascular disease have low (<10%) short-term (10 year) predicted risk but high lifetime predicted risk for coronary heart disease[30]
- Bariatric surgery reduces the relative risk for mortality by 40% in patients with history of cardiovascular events[31]
- Bariatric surgery reduces the number of cardiovascular deaths and events compared with usual care[32]
- American Heart Association Scientific Statement[33]: Bariatric surgery provides survival benefit[34-41] and is reserved for patients with severe obesity in whom medical therapy has failed and an acceptable operative risk is present

Emerging role for treatment of type-2 diabetes

- Resolution or improvement in clinical and biochemical markers of T2D in majority of bariatric surgery patients[42-44]
- 34.4% of patients undergoing RYGB, SG, or AGB procedures were "cured" at one year, according to the ADA definition: A1c <6%, FBG <100 mg/dL, without pharmacologic therapy or additional procedures[45, 46]

Criticisms

- No long-term strong evidence demonstrating acceptable safety and effectiveness; using relevant clinical outcome measures
- No RCT evidence for non-obese/overweight patients undergoing bariatric surgery specifically for T2DM
- No guidelines regarding the optimal procedure for patients with T2DM

4.2.2 Need for bariatric surgery

- Increasing prevalence of obesity
- Increasing distribution of obesity (geographic, socioeconomic, cultural)
- Recognition of obesity as a disease state requiring broader treatment and prevention strategies
- Recognition of pathophysiological association of obesity with T2DM, CVD, cancer, chronic debilitation, and other co-morbidities

4.2.3 Types of bariatric surgery

(see also summary of bariatric surgical procedures →106)

Purely malabsorptive bariatric surgery: reduces caloric absorption

Jejunal–ileal bypass (JIB; pure malabsorptive)

- First performed in 1952-1954 and popularized through the 1960s and 1970s
- Joining proximal small intestine to distal ileum
- Complications: blind loop syndrome, abdominal bloating, migratory arthralgias, hepatopathy, anal burning, fluid and electrolyte derangements, protein depletion, calcium/vitamin D deficiencies, nephrolithiasis, cholelithiasis, B12 deficiency, worse quality of life
- Replaced by more effective and safer procedures in mid-1970s

Combined restrictive and malabsorptive

Biliopancreatic diversion (BPD; combined)

- Developed by Scopinaro and colleagues in mid-1970s in Italy
- Partial distal gastrectomy, closure of duodenal stump, jejunum divided 250 cm proximal to ileocecal valve, distal (Roux; alimentary) limb anastomosed to proximal stomach, proximal (biliopancreatic) limb anastomosed to ileum 50 cm proximal to ileocecal valve
- Bile and gastropancreatic secretions prevent bacterial overgrowth and blind loop syndrome in biliopancreatic limb
- 200 cm Roux limb and 50 cm common channel
- 75% loss of excess weight in the first year
- 98% T2D cure in 10 years
- Improvement in hypertension and hyperlipidemia
- Significant long-term adverse effects: diarrhea, foul-smelling stool, flatulence, anemia, stomal ulceration, protein depletion, dumping, peripheral neuropathy, B12 deficiency and Wernicke encephalopathy, bone loss

- Therapies to address protein malnutrition:
  - Parenteral nutrition
  - ↑ gastric volume
  - Roux limb lengths increased to 300-350 cm

BPD with duodenal switch (BPDDS; combined)

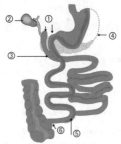

1. Duodenal switch
2. Gallbladder
3. Bilio pancreatic limb
4. Partially resected stomach
5. Digestive loop
6. Common loop

- Developed in the 1980s by Hess and colleagues
- Addresses morbidities with Scopinaro BPD
- Preserve pylorus to control gastric emptying and reduce dumping
- Preserve proximal duodenum to neutralize gastric acid and reduce stomal ulcerations
- Partial gastrectomy converted to sleeve configuration to keep pylorus intact
- Jejunum division at 40% of small bowel (ligament of Treitz to ileocecal valve) measured retrograde from the valve
- Longer common channel: 75-100 cm
- Roux limb: 250-300 cm

Roux-en-Y gastric bypass (RYGB; combined)

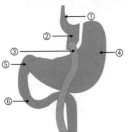

1. Esophagus
2. Proximal Pouch of stomach
3. "Short" Intestinal Roux Limb
4. Bypassed Portion of Stomach
5. Pylorus
6. Duodenum

- Developed by Mason and colleagues in mid-1960s and gained popularity in the late 1970s with further modifications
- Gastric restriction is the predominant feature
- Based on observation of patients having partial gastrectomy as part of Billroth II gastrojejunostomy for peptic ulcer disease lost weight
- Gastric pouch <30 mL (larger pouches would have greater wall tension [Laplace's Law] and therefore be more prone to dilate); modified to lesser curvature of upper stomach
- Roux-en-Y configuration replaces the standard loop gastrojejunostomy: less tension on jejunal loop, no bile reflux into pouch, malabsorptive
- Standard roux limb 100 cm; modified to >150 cm for patients with BMI >50 kg/m^2
- Less adverse effects, less weight loss, more weight regain, more dumping and marginal ulcers than BPDDS; still with significant calcium, iron, and B12 malabsorption resulting in bone loss and anemia

Purely restrictive bariatric surgery: Reduces volume of food that can be consumed

Gastroplasty

- Developed in 1970s and 1980s to avoid morbidities of malabsorptive procedures
- Vertical stapled pouch but staple line dehiscence and dilatation limited use
- Horizontal gastroplasty-gastric partitioning but pouch dilatation were still a problem
- Vertical banded gastroplasty based on theory that lesser curvature pouches resistant to dilatation; ideal pouch size <50 cm; staple line dehiscence and weight regain were still a problem

Gastric band

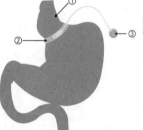

1. Small Stomach pouch
2. Adjustable gastric band
3. Port

- First performed by Wilkinson and Peloso in 1978 (nonadjustable)
- Least invasive bariatric procedure
- Early attempts unsuccessful due to slippage, prolapse, erosions, strictures
- Adjustable banding improved outcomes
- Less and slower weight loss compared with other bariatric procedures

Sleeve gastrectomy

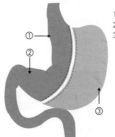

1. Gastric sleeve
2. Pylorus
3. Excised stomach

- Developed in late 1980s as standalone Magenstrasse and Mill procedure; and as part of the BPDDS by Marceau and colleagues in 1990s
- Resects excluded stomach-irreversible
- Vertical gastrectomy leaving narrow gastric tube preserving antrum and pylorus
- Smaller bougie size (32-French) associated with better weight loss
- Staple line leaks, stricture and gastric fistulas are minimized by modifications to the stapling technique
- May be a staging procedure, eventually leading to BPDDS or RYGB
- Technically less demanding, no foreign materials, less long-term problems (dumping, ulcers, hernias, nutrient deficiencies)

Laparoscopic approaches to bariatric procedures

- First performed in early 1990s
- Shorter length of stay
- Quicker recovery
- Less pain
- Less wound-related complications
- Similar benefits
- Learning curve requirement; more laparoscopic bariatric procedures now, compared with open procedures

New procedural technologies to treat obesity

- Endoscopic staplers and restriction devices
- Laparo-endoscopic single site
- Single-incision laparoscopic surgery
- Single-port access
- Natural orifice transluminal endoscopic surgery (NOTES)
- Fully robotic
- Hybrid robotic-laparoscopic

Summary of bariatric surgical procedures*

Procedure	Weight loss (%EBW)	Diabetes remission (%)	Morbidity**	Mortality***
VBG	5 y: 25-65	75-83	40-60	<1
AGB	10 y: 14-60	40-47	5	<1
SG	5 y: 58-62	66-91	11	<1
RYGB	10 y: 25-68	83-92	15	<1
BPDDS	10 y: 60-80	95-100	26	<1

* Laparoscopic procedures are preferred, ** 1-year morbidity,
*** 30-day postoperative mortality

VBG - Vertical Banded Gastroplasty, ABG - Adjustable Gastric Banding, SG - Sleeve Gastrectomy, RYGB - Roux-en-Y Gastric Bypass, BPDDS - Biliopancreatic Diversion with Duodenal Switch

4.2.4   Mechanisms of action of bariatric procedures

Restrictive

LAGB

- May limit patients to small meal size but this concept has been challenged
- Slows supra-band stomach emptying into the distal stomach
- No effect on overall gastric emptying
- Activates a peripheral satiety mechanism
- ↑ ghrelin proportionate to weight loss

SG (alone, as staged procedure, or BPDDS)

- ↓ production of the orexigenic hormone ghrelin with gastric fundus removal
- ↑ meal stimulated PYY comparable to changes with RYGB due to duodenal nutrient sensing and less digested chyme presenting to the L cells
- Less marked increases in meal-stimulated GLP-1

Gastric pouch (RYGB)

Variable effects on ghrelin but early short-term effects may be decreased due to vagal nerve manipulation during surgery and pouch configuration; later effects influenced by weight, insulin resistance, and individual differences

Malabsorptive and other mechanisms (neural, incretin)

RYGB

- "Taste" = chemical sensation of taste and olfaction plus oral perception of texture
- Taste receptors in mouth and small intestine
- Taste affects appetite, autonomic function, and insulin response
- Variable sense of taste for sweets; decreased pleasure (taste hedonics) with high-fat meats, high-calorie carbohydrates, milk, and ice cream
- Dumping produces avoidance behavior for decreased intake of sweets and fats but does not affect taste
- Intolerance of low-fat foods due to change in texture and altered intestinal transit and digestion
- ↑ basal and postprandial L cell GLP-1 and PYY secretion (anorexigenic and affects taste responses)
- Early weight independent increase in glucose stimulated oxyntomodulin (from L cells)
- Unclear fluctuations in bypassed duodenal meal-stimulated glucose-dependent insulinotropic peptide (GIP)
- Variable gut adaptation: ↑ bowel width, villus height, crypt depth, crypt proliferation
- Accelerated gastric emptying to liquids, slower gastric emptying with solids, and rapid intestinal transit
- ↓ leptin levels independent of ↓ adiposity
- Alteration in the gut flora and microbiome
- Unproven effects on energy expenditure in humans (increases in EE observed in animal models)

4.2.5 Indications

Weight loss

Current criteria

Overall:
- BMI criteria need to be adjusted downward for patients of Asian ethnic origin
- BMI ≥40 kg/m^2
- BMI ≥35 kg/m^2 and one obesity-related comorbidity
- BMI ≥30 kg/m^2 and T2D with high risk for cardiometabolic disease

Reimbursability:
- DRG morbid obesity code 278.01
- Reimbursement varies according to third party payer
- Centers for Medicare and Medicaid Services (CMS):
  - National Coverage Decision (NCD; CAG 00250R; 2006) limits bariatric surgery to centers accredited by the American College of Surgeons (ACS) or American Society for Metabolic and Bariatric Surgery (ASMBS)
  - NCD expands coverage to the LAGB (ICD-9 44.95; adjustment V53.51), ORYGB (44.39), LRYGB (44.38), OBPDDS or LBPDDS (44.68, 44.69, 43.89)
- SG remains as "noncovered procedure" by CMS NCD but now has a procedure code ICD 43.82 (laparoscopic) and 43.89 (open) grouped to DRG 619, 620 and 621 operative procedures for obesity

General statements
- Laparoscopic procedures preferred
- Patient preferences are incorporated into the decision making
- Available surgical expertise with certain procedures can affect procedure selection
- AGB: This is a lower risk procedure for patients expected to adhere with frequent follow-up as needed for band adjustment and mild (BMI 30-35 kg/m^2) to moderate (BMI 35-40 kg/m^2) obesity and relatively lower cardiometabolic risk
- SG: As a potential stand alone procedure for patients with relatively lower cardiometabolic risk with mild to moderate obesity or with severe (BMI ≥40 kg/m^2) obesity or relatively higher cardiometabolic risk as a staged procedure to be followed by an intestinal diversionary procedure
- RYGB: For patients with relatively higher cardiometabolic risk and/or severe obesity
- BDS-DS: This is a higher risk procedure for patients with severe obesity and high cardiometabolic risk in whom adherence with multiple nutritional supplements is expected

Diabetes

- In 2011 about 366 million people with T2D and expected to increase to about 522 million in 2030
- >60% patients with T2D are obese
- Only about 1/3 of patients treated according to standardized algorithms with lifestyle and pharmacotherapy achieve good glycemic control
- Intensifying pharmacotherapy can increase the risk for hypoglycemia and weight gain
- Therefore, there is a need for a surgical option in higher risk, recalcitrant patients with T2D
- Patients with BMI ≥35 kg/m^2 and T2D are already eligible for consideration for bariatric surgery
- Patients with BMI 30-35 kg/m^2 with T2D and other comorbidities cannot be controlled with optimal medical therapy may be considered for bariatric surgery
- Bariatric procedures (LAGB, SG, RYGB, and BPDDS) associated with improved endpoints (A1c <7%; LDL <100 mg/dL; sBP <130 mm Hg) as well as reduced cardiac events
- Omentectomy or liposuction: no effect on T2D
- T2D remission associated with:
  - Duration of T2D <5 years
  - No insulin requirement preoperatively
  - Postoperative weight loss
  - Maintenance of weight loss
  - Shift from high to low glycemic index foods
- Earlier surgical intervention may prevent pancreatic lipotoxicity and beta-cell damage

Mechanisms

- Proximal (foregut): Early nutrient proximal small bowel stimulation (SG, RYGB, BPDDS, DJB) due to rapid sleeve emptying affects incretin response; exclusion of chyme from the proximal small intestine
- Distal (hindgut): early nutrient distal small bowel stimulation (RYGB, BPDDS, SGIT) affects incretin response
- Ghrelin: resolutions with SG (coupled with salutary changes in GLP-1 and PYY)
- Other: significant weight loss (all procedures)

Investigational procedures

- Duodenojejunal bypass (DJB) with or without SG
- SG with ileal transposition (SGIT)
- Intragastric balloon
- Duodenal-jejunal bypass liner
- Electrophysiological (gastric stimulator) devices

Controversies

- Long-term data risks/benefits
- Surrogates versus outcomes
- Standardized definitions for diabetes improvements and remissions
- Standardized patient eligibility and selection criteria; including the creation of risk scores and modifying criteria away from simple BMI and A1c criteria

4.2.6   Preoperative management

Checklist

- Comprehensive medical history and physical examination
- Special attention to obesity-related comordities and factors that could affect a recommendation for bariatric surgery
- Aggressive case finding for rare causes of obesity are guided by historical and physical findings
- Routine chemistries, urinalysis, prothrombin time (INR), blood type, CBC
- Document the medical necessity for bariatric surgery

Cardiology and vascular medicine

- At least an EKG should be performed
- Additional testing guided by risk factors
- Formal cardiology consultation if there is known heart disease
- Continued use of beta-blockers associated with fewer cardiac events and 90-day mortality and should be considered in patients at risk for heart disease
- Diagnostic evaluation for deep venous thrombosis (DVT) for history of cor pulmonale or previous DVT

Pulmonary

- Chest x-ray
- Routine pre-operative screening for obstructive sleep apnea, which is associated with increased all cause mortality with bariatric surgery; confirmatory polysomnography if screening tests positive
- Additional testing guided by risk factors
- Formal pulmonary consultation, and arterial blood gas measurements, for a history of intrinsic lung disease or disordered sleep patterns
- Smoking cessation at any time before bariatric surgery; preferably at least 6-8 weeks preoperatively

Nutritional evaluation

- Evaluate ability to incorporate nutritional and eating behavior changes before and after surgery
- Pre-operative bariatric surgery patients frequently have nutritional deficiencies and should have an appropriate nutritional evaluation
- B12, D, iron deficiencies are frequent before and after surgery and should be checked
- B1, RBC folate, homocysteine, methylmalonic acid, and other nutrient markers should be checked if clinically indicated

Endocrine/metabolic

- Optimize glycemic control:
  - Diabetes comprehensive care plan
  - Healthy eating pattern
  - Medical nutrition therapy
  - Physical activity guidance
  - Pharmacotherapy as needed
- TSH is not indicated solely because a patient is obese
- Fasting lipid profile and standard management
- Prophylaxis for acute gouty attack with history of gout
- Routine bone density is not indicated

Reproductive

- Avoid pregnancy preoperatively
- Contraceptive counseling as needed
- Discontinue estrogen: 1 cycle of oral contraceptives in premenopausal women and 3 weeks of hormone replacement therapy in postmenopausal women
- Evaluation for polycystic ovary syndrome (PCOS) in women if clinically indicated; women with PCOS should be advised their fertility status may improve postoperatively

Gastrointestinal

- Cirrhosis or hepatomegaly associated with adverse outcomes and should be evaluated
- Consider 10% weight loss over 2 weeks with energy restricted diets to ↓ hepatic volume
- GI symptoms to be evaluated by endoscopy and/or barium studies
- Gallbladder evaluation as clinically indicated
- Routine H. pylori screening in high prevalence areas

Cancer

Age and risk appropriate screening

Psychiatric

- Routine psycho-social evaluation
- Formal mental health evaluation for history of substance abuse or poorly controlled psychiatric illness
- Identification of loss-of-control eating patterns can assist with procedure selection
- Limit alcohol consumption; high-risk patients (RYGB, BPDDS) to avoid alcohol due to impaired alcohol metabolism

Insurance clearance

- Financial counseling
- Bariatric surgery program to facilitate with third-party payer

Informed consent

- Dynamic process
- Thorough discussion of risks and benefits
- Procedural options
- Surgeon choice and experience with specific procedures
- Medical institution choice and accreditation
- Provide educational materials and sessions

Bariatric surgery team

- Bariatric surgeon
- Bariatric coordinator
- Internist with nutrition or obesity medicine experience
- Registered dietitian
- Psychologist/psychiatrist
- Medical consultants as needed: Endocrinologist, cardiologist, pulmonologist/ sleep medicine, physical medicine and rehabilitation
- Administration:
- Social worker; financial counselor

4.2.7 Early postoperative management

RD supervision of a protocol-derived, staged meal progression based on the specific procedure

Stage 1	POD 1-2 clears, no sugar, caffeine, or carbonation
Stage 2	POD 3 clears, salty fluids, solid liquids, sugar-free ice pops, the full high protein liquids, low sugar, nonfat dairy
Stage 3	POD 10-14 increase liquids and then soft protein sources with 4-6 small meals/day; avoid drinking liquids with meals and use small plates and utensils; at 4 weeks to add well-cooked soft vegetables and peeled fruits, eat protein first; no rice, bread, past until protein can be consumed; at 5 weeks to add salads; adequate hydration; higher priority to consume >60 g supplemental protein/day and maintain stage 3 for up to 12 weeks with BPDDS
Stage 4	About 6 weeks postop, increase food to targets based on BMI and age; chew small bites of food thoroughly; at least 5 daily servings of fresh fruits and vegetables; try to eliminate concentrated sweets to minimize dumping and reduce caloric intake; consume sufficient fluids at least 30 min after meals to avoid underhydration and dumping

Nutritional

- Chewable or liquid nutrient supplements
- 2 multivitamins a day
- Iron with vitamin C (40-65 mg/day)
- Calcium citrate (1200-1500 mg elemental calcium in divided doses)
- Vitamin D (at least 3000 units/day and then titrated to 25-hydroxyvitamin D levels >30 ng/mL); in recalcitrant cases (usually BPDDS), may need as high as 50,000 units a day with concurrent calcitriol dosing
- Vitamin B12 orally (at least 350 mcg/day), sublingual, intranasal (500 mcg q week), subcutaneous, or intramuscular (1000 mcg/month or 3000 mcg q 6 months) to maintain sufficient levels (may not be needed in patients with LAGB who were replete preoperatively)
- For BPDDS: "ADEK" supplements (vitamin A 4000 IU, cholecalciferol 400 IU, vitamin E 150 IU,vitamin K 0.15 mg)
- Modular protein may be needed after malabsorptive procedures
- Nutrition support (enteral and/or parenteral) should be considered in any patient at high nutritional risk and unable to meet their needs for 5-7 days (noncritical illness) or 3-7 days (critical illness)

Glycemic (in patients with T2D)

- Fasting blood glucose determinations periodically
- Self monitoring of blood glucose at home, preprandial and postprandial depending on glycemic status
- Discontinue sulfonylureas and meglitinides
- Typically continue metformin initially
- May consider incretin-based therapies for patients who are not meeting glycemic targets
- If taking insulin, adjust to avoid hypoglycemia
- Hold all anti-diabetes medications if T2D is in remission

Other nonsurgical

- ICU or monitored telemetry for first 24-48 hours after surgery for known coronary artery disease or high perioperative risk
- Aggressive pulmonary toilet, incentive spirometry, oxygen supplementation, early continuous positive airway pressure (CPAP) as indicated
- DVT prophylaxis: sequential compression devices, sq heparin; extended chemoprophylaxis after hospital discharge in high-risk patients
- Early ambulation
- Evaluate for acute postoperative complication in patients with respiratory distress, failure to wean from mechanical ventilation, hemodynamic changes, or possibly elevated C-reactive protein:
  - Exclude pulmonary embolus
  - Upper GI gastrografin study for anastomotic leak; if high suspicion, then exploratory laparotomy/laparoscopy
  - Consider gastrografin study in absence of abnormal signs/symptoms to exclude subclinical leaks before hospital discharge
- Check creatine kinase (CK) levels in patients suspected to have rhabdomyolysis

4.2.8 Late postoperative management

Follow-up

- To monitor for surgical complications, nonsurgical complications, nutritional status, and weight loss progress; band adjustments with AGB
- AGB: every month for first 6 months and then 1-2 times a year thereafter
- RYGB/BPDDS: every 1-3 months for the first 6-12 months and then 1-2 times a year thereafter

Dietetic

- Evaluate for maladaptive eating behaviors
- Review healthy eating patterns

Laboratory monitoring

- SG/RYGB: CBC, basic metabolic panel, glucose, liver function, iron, TIBC, ferritin, vitamin B12, lipid profile, 25-OH vitamin D (optional: intact PTH, thiamine, RBC folate, methylmalonic acid, homocysteine)
- BPDDS: CBC, comprehensive metabolic, glucose, iron, TIBC, ferritin, vitamin B12, albumin, prealbumin, liver function, RBC folate (optional: methylmalonic acid, homocysteine), vitamin A, 25-OH vitamin D, Vitamin E, vitamin K1, INR, intact PTH, 24 hour urine calcium, 24 hour urine oxalate, zinc, selenium (consider: thiamine, selenium, zinc, carnitine, fatty acid chromatography)

Nutritional deficiency

- AGB: monitor iron, B12, and folate status and replete as needed
- SG/RYGB: monitor iron, B12, folate, calcium, D, copper, and zinc status and replete as needed
- BPDDS: monitor protein, iron, B12, folate, calcium, vitamins ADEK, copper, and zinc status and replete as needed
- Additional nutrients to monitor based on clinical signs and symptoms: essential fatty acid, selenium
- Vitamin C therapy may be added to augment iron absorption
- Intravenous iron may be necessary in recalcitrant iron deficiency states
- Thiamine deficiency should be suspected in patients with rapid weight loss, severe and chronic vomiting, excessive alcohol use, neuropathy/encephalopathy, or heart failure, and should be replaced intravenously and then orally
- Selenium deficiency should be suspected if anemia, fatigue, persistent diarrhea, cardiomyopathy
- Zinc deficiency should be suspected if hair loss and rash

Gastrointestinal

- Nausea, vomiting, abdominal pain, and diarrhea need to be evaluated
- Avoid nonsteroidal anti-inflammatory drugs since they are associated with anastomotic ulcerations and perforations
- Persistent vomiting, regurgitation, or obstructive symptoms after AGB should be managed with immediate removal of fluid from the band
- Persistent gastro-esophageal reflux, regurgitation, cough, or aspiration pneumonia may represent an excessively tight band and necessitate referral back to the surgeon
- Prophylactic cholecystectomy may be considered with RYGB to prevent gallstones; in those patients without cholecystectomy, oral ursodeoxycholic acid may be used
- After BPDDS, bacterial overgrowth in biliopancreatic limb can be treated with metronidazole or rifaximin; probiotics containing Lactobacillus plantarum 299v and Lactobacillus GG may be considered in recalcitrant cases
- After RYGB/BPDDS, severe abdominal pain requires abdominal and pelvic CT to exclude bowel obstruction

Non-insulinoma pancreatogenous hypoglycemia syndrome (NIPHS)

- RYGB or BPDDS
- Postprandial symptoms
- Differential diagnosis: factitious, iatrogenic, dumping, insulinoma
- Treatment: octreotide, diazoxide, acarbose, and/or calcium-channel antagonists; or surgery (gastric restriction, partial/total pancreatectomy)

Physical activity

- Moderate aerobic 150-300 min a week
- Strength training 2-3 times a week

Bone

- In RYGB/BPDDS: dual X-ray absorptiometry (DXA) at baseline and two years (can use forearm DXA imaging if too heavy for conventional DXA tables)
- Consider IV bisphosphonates (eg, zolendronic acid, 5 mg annually) in patients with osteoporosis once vitamin D levels are replete

Kidney stones

- Higher risk after malabsorptive procedures (RYGB, BPDDS)
- Monitor 24 hour urinary oxalate, citrate, calcium, uric acid
- Avoid dehydration
- If oxalate stones or high urinary oxalate:
  - Low oxalate diet
  - Consider oral calcium and potassium citrate therapy
  - Consider probiotics containing Oxalobacter formigenes

Precautions

- Avoid pregnancy for 12-18 months postoperatively; counseling regarding non-oral contraceptives; if pregnant after LAGB, band adjustments as needed for appropriate weight gain for fetal health
- Lipid-lowering agents should not be stopped unless clearly indicated
- Anti-hypertensive agents should not be stopped unless clearly indicated, though dose adjustments may be needed
- Avoid tobacco use to improve wound healing and avoid anastomotic ulcers
- Ongoing support groups

Surgical

- Weight regain, inadequate weight loss, or severe complications may require revision surgery; if not responsive to revision, then reversal procedures should be considered
- Abdominal wall hernias:
  - Asymptomatic - can wait until weight loss has stabilized and nutritional status improved (usually 12-18 months after surgery)
  - Symptomatic - prompt surgical evaluation
- Body contouring surgery should be considered 12-18 months after surgery to manage excess tissue that impairs hygiene, causes discomfort, and/or is disfiguring

List of references

22 Zhao The gut microbiota and obesity: from corretlion to causality. L Nat Rev Microbiol 2013 Aug 16;11(9):639-47.
23 Kushner R. Practical Manual of Clinical Obesity. Wiley-Blackwell 2013
24 Li Z et al. Meta-analysis: pharmacologic treatment of obesity: Ann Intern Med 2005142:532-6
25 J Clin Endocrinol Metab. 2011 Oct;96(10):3067-77. Epub 2011 Jul 27.A one-year randomized trial of lor-caserin for weight loss in obese and overweight adults: the BLOSSOM trial. Fidler MC, Sanchez M, Rae-ether B, Weissman NJ, Smith SR, Shanahan WR, Anderson CM; BLOSSOM Clinical Trial Group
26 Gadde KM et al. Lancet. 2011 Apr 16;377(9774):1341-52. Epub 2011 Apr 8. Effects of low-dose, control-led-release, phentermine plus topiramate combination on weight and associated comorbidities in over-weight and obese adults (CONQUER): a randomised, placebo-controlled, phase 3 trial
27 Garvey WT et al. Am J Clin Nutr. 2012 Feb;95(2):297-308. Epub 2011 Dec 7.Two-year sustained weight loss and metabolic benefits with controlled-release phentermine/topiramate in obese and overweight adults (SEQUEL): a randomized, placebo-controlled, phase 3 extension study
28 Logue J, et al. BMJ 2010; 340: 474-477
29 Mechanick JI et al. AACE/TOS/ASMBS Guidelines Clinical Practice Guidelines for the Perioperative Nutritional, Metabolic, and Nonsurgical Support of the Bariatric Surgery Patientâ?"2013 Update: Cosponsored by American Association of Clinical Endocrinologists, The Obesity Society, and American Society for Metabolic & Bariatric Surgery. Surgery for Obesity and Related Diseases9(2013)159-191.
30 Mackey RH et al. Am J Cardiol 2012; PMID 22742719
31 Johnson RJ et al. Am Surg 2012; 78: 685-692
32 Sjostrom L et al. JAMA 2012; 307: 56-65
33 Poirier P, et al. Circulation 2011; 123: 1683-1701
34 Adams TD, et al. N Engl J Med 2007; 357: 753-761
35 Sjostrom L, et al. N Engl J Med 2007; 357:741-752
36 MacDonald KG Jr, et al. J Gastroint Surg 1997; 1: 213-220
37 Sowemimo OA, et al. Surg Obes Relat Dise 2007; 3: 73- 77
38 Christou NV, et al. Ann Surg 2004; 240: 416-423
39 Busetto L, et al. Surg Obes Relat Dis 2007; 3: 496-502
40 Flum DR, et al. J Am Coll Surg 2004; 199: 543-551
41 Peeters A, et al. Ann Surg 2007; 1028-1033
42 Buchwald H, et al. Am J Med 2009; 122: 248-256
43 Mingrone G, et al. N Engl J Med 2012; 366: 1577-1585
44 Schauer PR, et al. N Engl J Med 2012; 366: 1567-1576
45 Poumaras DJ, et al. Br J Surg 2012; 99: 100-103
46 Buse JB, Diabetes Care 2009; 32: 2133-2135

5 Nutrition Support

5.1 Enteral Nutrition Support

5.1.1 Definition

Complete nutrition delivered to the stomach or proximal small bowel in patients unable to meet nutritional needs with oral nutrition alone

5.1.2 Indications

Functional GI tract and one of the following

- Insufficient oral intake to meet nutritional needs with history and expected duration of impairment >1-10 days (time dependent on inflammation and clinical judgment:
  - Critical illness 1-3 days
  - Noncritical illness with inflammation 5-7 days
  - Simple starvation without inflammation 7-10 days
- Neuro-psychiatric function:
  - Impaired appetite (anorexia syndromes)
  - Impaired food-seeking behavior
- Aerodigestive tract disorder:
  - Dysphagia
  - Esophageal dysmotility
  - Gastric dysmotility
  - Obstruction (oropharynx to stomach)
  - Other anatomical or functional impairments
- Increased demands (exceeding capability of oral nutrition):
  - Burns
  - Trauma
  - Wounds
  - Critical illness
- Severe malnutrition:
  - Preoperative management
  - Unresponsive to oral nutrition

5.1.3   Contraindications

- Intestinal obstruction (distal to potential feeding jejunostomy placement)
- Intractable vomiting
- Intractable diarrhea (unresponsive to elemental formulas and aggressive anti-diarrheal therapy)
- Short bowel syndrome (usually in association with <100 cm small bowel with intact colon and <150 cm without intact colon)
- Intestinal dysmotility syndromes:
  - Paralytic ileus (narcotics or postoperative)
  - Neuropathic
  - Idiopathic
- Distal high output fistula that can't be bypassed with enteral device placement
- Severe GI bleed
- Anticipation of frequent enteral nutrition interruptions:
  - Procedural
  - Other logistics (eg, tube feeding availability, pump malfunction)

5.1.4   Practical benefits
Practical benefits relative to the use of parenteral nutrition benefits

- Stimulates gallbladder
- Trophic for commensal intestinal bacteria and normal microbiome
- Maintains nominal gut immunity
- Maintains nominal intestinal mucosal integrity:
  - Villus crypt depth
  - Tight junctions
  - Paracrine communication
  - Molecular/cellular signaling
- ↑ gut protein synthesis
- Maintains nominal absorptive function
- Reduces bacterial translocation and risk for systemic infection
- Potential for cost savings

5.1.5 Risks

- Related to placement, insertion, surgery, endoscopy or other procedural events
- Discomfort in some patients with NG tube
- Nausea, regurgitation, vomiting, aspiration, and possible aspiration pneumonia
- Tube dislodgement
- Infection:
  - Dermatitis at percutaneous stoma site
  - Sinusitis with nasogastric tube
  - Cutaneous or intra-abdominal with surgical gastrostomy or jejunostomy tube placement
- Erosion of nasal-pharyngeal tract with prolonged NG tube placement
- Perforation and leaks
- Gastric or hepatic with percutaneous endoscopic or surgical placement

5.1.6 Feeding tubes

Nasogastric	Flexible small bore tube preferred (for days to weeks of use)
Orogastric	• Commonly used in newborns • In adults may be used for intubated patients or patients in whom NGT is contraindicated
Trans- or Postpyloric	• With gastric dysmotility • Anatomical abnormalities precluding gastric placement

Gastrostomy	• Percutaneous (PEG):
	  – Antibiotic prophylaxis decreases risk of peristomal infection[47]
	  – Staphylococcus aureus is most common organism
	  – Consider cefazolin 1 g IV, ceftriaxone 1 g IV or amoxicillin-clavulanic acid 1.2 g IV x 1 30 min pre-procedure
	• Surgical gastrostomy (G tube)

Jejunostomy (J tube)	• Feeding should be below the Ligament of Treitz if 2 or more risk factors:
	  – Prior aspiration
	  – Decreased level of consciousness
	  – Neuromuscular disease
	  – Structural abnormalities of aerodigestive tract
	  – Endotracheal intubation
	  – Vomiting
	  – Persistently high gastric residual volume (GRV)
	  – Need for supine positioning

5.1.7   Choosing a formula
Standard formulas
Intact/whole protein

Sources: casein, soy, whey

Range 1.0–2.0 kcal/cc

Use calorie dense for patients who require volume restriction or for cycled feeds over shorter time periods

Fiber-containing

- Fructooligosaccharide (FOS) fermented by colonic bacteria to short-chain fatty acid (SCFA) provides energy source for colonocytes
- Soluble fiber (pectin, guar) ↑ colonic sodium and water absorption and may help with diarrhea
- Insoluble fiber (soy polysaccharide) ↑ fecal weight and ↓ fecal transit time:
  - Viscous use is limited; does not improve glucose control

Renal disease

- Electrolyte restricted- lower phosphorus, magnesium, potassium, sodium
- Concentrated to reduce volume and free water (usually 1.8 kcal/cc)
- Higher protein for those on renal replacement therapy (RRT)
- Lower protein for those not on RRT
- Higher proportion of essential amino acids as nitrogen source
- Higher concentration of carnitine

Liver disease

- ↑ branched-chain amino acid (BCAA) and ↓ aromatic and sulphur-containing amino acids
- May improve some forms of hepatic encephalopathy

Diabetes

- Higher fat, lower carbohydrate
- Carbohydrate modifications:
  - Additional fiber and FOS; Altered maltodextrins with resistant glucose-glucose linkages that retard intestinal digestion
- Result in lower peak glucose, lower glycemic variability, lower insulin requirements, improved markers of glycemic control (eg, A1c and average glucose levels)
- ↑ monounsaturated fatty acids (MUFA; replaces some of the carbohydrate calories)- ↓ postprandial glucose, insulin, and triglycerides
- Usually with ↑ chromium

Pulmonary disease

- Based on premise and limited data that the respiratory quotient (CO_2 production) is directly related to the carbohydrate:fat ratio (not a consistent finding in all clinical studies; rather, CO_2 production is more related to total calories in some studies)
- Higher fat, lower carbohydrate formulas
- For ARDS: Formulas rich in gamma linolenic and eicosapentanoic acids may reduce ventilator time and improve surrogate markers (eg, inflammation and pulmonary function)

Critically ill

- Use fiber free formula to:
  - Avoid slower gastric emptying
  - Avoid increased risk of bowel obstruction
- Prefer (semi-) elemental formula
- Modular arginine (3 g/day):
  - May be conditionally essential during periods of stress due to increased requirements
  - Routine use is controversial
  - Purported benefits for wound healing, optimizing nitrogen retention, infectious complications, and overall clinical outcomes
  - May increase mortality in sepsis SIRS patients
- Glutamine:
  - May be conditionally essential during periods of stress due to increased requirements
  - Can modulate immune function and proteolysis
  - Supplementation with glutamine may lead to ↓ in nosocomial infections in patients with systemic inflammatory response and a ↓ in pneumonia, sepsis, and bacteremia in trauma patients[48]
- Omega 3 fatty acids:
  - Reduces mortality, secondary infection, and lOS in patients with SIRS and ARDS[49]
  - May be associated with platelet dysfunction and bleeding
- Nucleic acids:
  - Play role in ATP metabolism and modulation of immune function
  - Deficiency may develop during critical illness
  - Immune enhancing formulas containing nucleotides have been shown to reduce infections, ventilator days and LOS for critically ill and postsurgical patients but not proven to be isolated effect[50]
  - Evidence base is not conclusive

Burn patients

- Use high protein, high calorie formula due to increased metabolic demands and nitrogen requirements that may exceed 2.0-2.5 g/kg/day
- Glutamine decreases infection and length of stay (LOS)[51]

Post-operative GI surgery patients

Glutamine may be beneficial

5.1.8   Immunonutrition

Glutamine	• Amino acid with tropic effects on the small intestine mucosa • Helps restore integrity of GI mucosa and ↓ bacterial trans-location
Arginine	• Precursor of nitric oxide and hydroxyproline important for connective tissue repair • Essential substrate for immune cells especially lymphocyte function • Requirements increase during periods of stress
Omega 3 fatty acids	• EPA and DHA alter membrane structure and function and gene transcription • Anti-inflammatory properties through incorp. in membrane structure and function, suppression of proinflammatory transcription factors, modulation of eicosanoid production • May suppress inflammatory response and capillary leakage • Its products may benefit wound healing
Gamma linoleic acid (GLA) omega 6 lipid from borage oil	Synergistic with EPA and DHA in ↓ inflammation and organ injury
Prebiotics	• Selective stimulation of growth and/or activity of one or more microbial species in the gut microbiota that confer health benefits to the host • Typically inulin-type fructans (inulin, oligofructose, fructooligosaccharides [FOS]) • May ↑ fecal bifidobacteria • Fermentable fiber for colon health: may decrease risk of diarrhea
Probiotics	• Live microorganisms which when administered in adequate amounts confer a health benefit on the host • Eg, Lactobacilli, bifidobacteria, saccharomyces • May reduce diarrhea • Case reports of infection caused by probiotics: – Caution in immunosuppressed patients

5.1.9 Clinical outcomes[52]

Perioperative	• Early EN (6 hrs) reduces anastomotic inflammation in GI surgery patients
	• Immunonutrition may reduce infectious complications after GI and non-GI surgery:
	  – Supplemented arginine, omega 3 fatty acids, nucleotides before and after surgery
	  – Effective regardless of baseline nutritional status
	• Reduced infections

Cancer (excludes BMT)	No benefit to EN vs volitional nutrition support
Liver disease	• Does not improve morbidity or LOS • Survival benefit demonstrated with EN over no treatment
Pancreatic	• EN safer than PN • Associated with reduced risk of infectious complications • No difference between LOS vs no treatment
IBD	• No difference in remission rates with EN vs PN • Enteral nutrition is inferior to steroids in reducing inflammation
Critical illness	• EN reduces infection rate • No difference of days on vent with EN vs PN
Burn	Early EN reduces infection rate
AIDS	No difference in mortality, infectious complications, CD4 cell counts or quality of life with EN vs volitional nutrition support
Stroke	No difference in survival with early vs late EN (7 day)

5.1.10 Safety

• Confirm tube position
• Bacterial contamination:
  – Prefilled ready to hang closed systems
  – Hand washing
  – Cleansing top of cans before opening
  – Wearing gloves
  – Observe cut-off hang times
• Ensure tube stability

5.1.11 Initiation of feeding

- Dilution not necessary
- Begin full strength feed at low rate (10-30 cc/hr)
- Advance to goal over 24-48 hours
- Increase by 10-20 mL every 4-8 hours

5.1.12 Continuous feeding

- Administered via pump
- May be cycled over 10-20 hours or 24 hours
- Reasons to cycle feeds:
  - ↑ appetite during the day
  - Allow for increase daytime activity
- Provide flushes every 6 hours for 24 hours feeds
- Provide flushes before and after cycled feeds and every 6 hours in between

5.1.13 Bolus feeding

- Boluses 240-480 cc
- Initiate ½-1 can per feeding
- Syringe over 10-15 min
- Gravity over 30 min
- Provide flushes before and after each feeding

5.1.14 Prescribing flushes

- Flushes help prevent clogging and provide fluid requirements
- Estimate water requirements (typically 30-40 cc/kg/day; based on metabolic rate, body composition, and age):
  - Younger, more percentage of muscle: closer to 40
  - Older, less percentage of muscle: closer to 30
- Calculate water in formula provided (70%-80%, see above)
- Subtract provided from required
- Divide by number of flushes planned
- Use water in gastric feeding in patient with normal or high serum sodium
- Use ½ NS or NS with Jejunostomy feeds
- Use ½ NS or NS in hyponatremic patients

5.1.15 Gastric residual volumes

- Unreliable
- Does not predict aspiration pneumonia
- No standardization for actionable value (eg, 150-500 mL; 50% infused volume)
- Duration of time between assessments and clinical exam may be important

5.1.16 Treatment of delayed gastric emptying

- Discontinue narcotics
- Switch to low fat formula
- Switch to formula without fiber
- Switch to isotonic formula (if hypertonic)
- Correct hypovolemia
- Reduce rate of infusion
- Supplemental PN to meet nutritional needs in high-risk patients (eg, critical illness)
- Postpyloric tube placement
- Metoclopramide:
  - Inhibits dopamine action in the gut
  - ↑ antral and small intestinal motility
  - Dose: 10-20 mg QID
  - Can cause diarrhea

5.1.17 Mechanical complications

Mechanical complications of enteral access device

Occlusion

- Bicarbonate and pancreatic enzyme solution
- Warm water and gentle pressure
- Guide wire manipulation and agitation

Diarrhea[53]

Mechanisms

- ↑ water secretion into the colon
- Concomitant antibiotics
- Clostridium difficile and other pathogens with bacterial overgrowth
- Ischemic bowel
- Occult inflammatory bowel

Management

- Fiber may prevent diarrhea by reducing the rate of gastric emptying and improving gut barrier function and increasing colonic fluid and electrolyte absorption
- Fiber undergoes fermentation to SCFA that reverse the abnormal colonic water secretion
- Prebiotics and probiotics may suppress enteropathogenic colonization and minimize risk from antibiotics and C. difficile
- Evaluate for C. difficile
- Review medications:
  - Antibiotics
  - Syrup or liquid medications with high osmolar load or containing sorbitol leading to osmotic laxative effect
- Water and electrolyte replenishment
- Loperamide, loperamide oxide or codeine
- Consider adding soluble fiber
- Consider semi-elemental formula (with ↑ MCT and ↓ LCT)
- Avoid discontinuing EN:
  - To reduce risk of underfeeding
  - Bowel rest exacerbates bacterial overgrowth and GI dysmotility and ↑ risk of undernutrition
  - Consider supplemental PN (in higher risk patients)

Hypernatremia ("Tube feeding syndrome")

- Deamination and deamidation of amino acids yields ammonia and other nitrogenous metabolites requiring obligate renal free water excretion
- Common in critical illness, especially after cardiac surgery, due to concurrent:
  - Deliberate avoidance of fluid overload
  - Use of diuretics
  - Catecholamine-induced nephrogenic diabetes insipidus
- Higher risk with high protein formula
- Treat with increased free water flushes
- Consider diluting feeds 1/2 to 2/3 to 3/4 strength and increasing infusion rate to maintain same nutritional prescription
- Consider lower protein formula until corrected

5.1.18 Inadequate delivery of calories

- PEP uP protocol has been effective in improving nutrition delivered in ICU setting[54]:
  - Targets 24 hours volume rather than hourly rate
  - Nurses can make up volume if prior interruption of feeds for non-GI reasons
  - Protein supplements are provided at onset and then discontinued if EN is well tolerated to avoid protein deficit
  - Motility agents given when EN is started and then discontinued if not needed
  - Threshold GRV 250 mL

5.1.19 Monitoring

Weight	• 1-2 times per week • Daily in the intensive care unit
Electrolytes	• Serum Na, K, Mg, Phos, BUN • May need to increase or decrease free water provided based on serum Na • May need to change to or from electrolyte restricted formula based on renal function • Monitor daily until stable then periodically
Glucose	• Higher risk of hyperglycemia with EN than oral diet • Consider change to glycemia-targeted specialized nutrition/diabetes-specific formula and/or insulinized if hyperglycemia
Additional nutrient intake	• Assess continued need for nutrition support or need to adjust calories provided • If the oral intake is about 50% of requirements for 2-3 days, can decrease enteral nutrition
GI signs/symptoms of intolerance	• Abdominal distension • Abdominal pain • Nausea/vomiting • Diarrhea
Biochemical nutritional markers	• Serum albumin • Serum prealbumin • Nitrogen balance (UUN)

5.1.20 Medicare coverage for home enteral nutrition

- Enteral nutrition is considered reasonable and necessary for a patient with a functioning gastrointestinal tract who, due to pathology, or nonfunction of, the structures that normally permit food to reach the digestive tract, which can not maintain weight and strength commensurate with his or her general condition:
  - Eg, head and neck cancer with reconstructive surgery and central nervous system disease leading to interference with the neuromuscular mechanisms of ingestion of such severity that the beneficiary cannot be maintained with oral feeding
- Medical documentation (eg, hospital records, clinical findings from the attending physician) must permit an independent conclusion that the patient's condition meets the requirements of the prosthetic device benefit and that enteral nutrition therapy is medically necessary
- If the claim involves a pump, it must be supported by sufficient medical documentation to establish that the pump is medically necessary, ie, gravity feeding is not satisfactory due to aspiration, diarrhea, dumping syndrome

5.2 Parenteral Nutrition Support

5.2.1 Key principles

- To provide nutrients intravenously
- Generally in patients at high nutritional risk with nonfunctional, or uncertain, GI tracts
- Must be delivered in a safe fashion

5.2.2 Indications

Nonfunctional GI tract

- Obstruction
- Severe malabsorption
- Large chyle leak (chylothorax, chylous ascites)
- Distal intestinal fistula
- Paralytic ileus
- Bowel perforation
- Mesenteric ischemia
- Post major abdominal surgery NPO 5-10 days

Uncertain GI tract

Less severe forms of the above where the patient is still unable to meet nutritional needs with enteral nutrition alone

Inaccessible GI tract

- Anorexia and refusal to place enteral access
- Altered mental status and unable to place enteral access
- BIPAP, CPAP and inability to place access device
- Diseases of the aero-digestive tract and unable to place enteral access device:
  - Head and neck cancer
  - Trachea-esophageal fistula
  - Stomatitis, esophagitis, or other inflammation/infectious condition
  - Dysphagia
  - Zenker's diverticulum
  - Postoperative dysfunction
- Patient refusal for enteral access
- Physician refusal for enteral access
- Risks > benefits of enteral access

Inability to meet nutritional needs with enteral nutrition alone

- Anatomical
- Physiological
- Logistical:
  - Procedural interruptions
  - Nondelivery of nutritional product

Must be at high nutritional risk

- NRS 2002 ≥3
- NRI <83.5
- No nutrition for >3-5 days (critically ill)
- No nutrition for >5-7 days (noncritically ill)
- Anticipate high nutritional risk without PN implementation

Must be consistent with goals of care

5.2.3   Venous access devices

Peripheral

- Conventional catheter (general 1-3 inches and 20 gauge or smaller) in hand or forearm typically lasting 1-3 days. Used for peripheral PN (PPN).
- Midline catheter (3-10 inches [usually 8 inches] and 18 or 20 gauge) in brachial or cephalic veins with tip below the axillary line and typically last 1-6 weeks; used for PPN

Central

- Triple lumen catheter (TLC) is the most common catheter used in hospitals for administration of PN. They are percutaneously inserted into the internal or external jugular, subclavian or axillary, or femoral vein with tip in the superior vena cava or cavoatrial junction. The proximal (white) port is for medication and maintenance fluids, mid (blue) port for medication and can be dedicated for PN, and distal (brown; largest) port for blood transfusion or sampling, or medication if needed.
- Peripherally inserted central catheter (PICC; one or two lumen) are 25-60 cm in length for insertion with guide wire in the cephalic, basilic, or brachial vein and tip in the superior vena cava or cavoatrial junction. They are sutured in place and can last up to a year (usually 3-6 months or as needed). Usually used for home PN
- Hickman or Broviac (single or double lumen) indwelling catheter from chest wall site to entry in jugular and tip placed in superior vena cava or cavoatrial junction
- Groshung (single or double lumen) differs from Hickman or Broviac by having 3-way valve at tip that may reduce risk of clotting, air embolism, and blood reflux
- Portacath (single or double) medical appliance serving as a reservoir system implanted under the skin, usually placed in the upper chest. A catheter runs from the portal to the jugular vein, subclavian vein, or superior vena cava. The port is accessed with a 90° Huber point needle or winged needle; usually used for home PN

Dialysis catheters

Dialysis catheters are available for PN use but generally avoided due to risk of infection and desire not to lose dialysis access

5.2.4   Inspection of parenteral nutrition infusion

Pump

Depends on hospital and home PN vendor

Catheter care

- Dressing (occlusive or transparent): inspect for bleeding, infection, intactness
- Line connectors inspect for leaks
- Bag spike:inspect for leaks
- 1.2 micron filter (for PN with lipid) inspect for correct placement
- 0.2 micron filter (for PN without lipid) inspect for correct placement
- Ethanol lock therapy is an optional measure in attempt to reduce risk for infection primarily in home PN patients

PN destabilization of lipid emulsion/admixture increases risk for lipid emboli

- Can refrigerate before addition of vitamins for:
  - 2:1 up to 30 days
  - 3:1 up to 10 days
- Creaming: triglyceride particles accumulate at top of bag (benign and reversible with gentle agitation; if recurs in 1-2 hrs, then abort the infusion)
- Aggregation: triglyceride particles clumping throughout bag (immediately discard)
- Coalescence: triglyceride particles fuse into large particles (immediately discard)
- Cracking: frank separation of lipid from aqueous components of the emulsion, (immediately discard)

5.2.5   Formulation

Nomenclature

Parenteral- not through the gastrointestinal tract; intravenous:
- **Total parenteral nutrition (TPN)**: generally a misnomer since it may not provide all nutritional requirements; this always refers to a central venous PN formula that cannot infuse via a peripheral venous catheter
- **Peripheral parenteral nutrition (PPN):** can infuse via peripheral or central catheter since the osmolarity is constrained to a lower amount
  - Should only be used if PN not expected for more than 10-14 days and providing that the patient can maintain sufficient peripheral venous access for the PPN and other IV meds:
  - 2:1 PPN maximum Osm = 800 mOsm/kg
  - 3:1 PPN maximum Osm = 900 mOsm/kg
  - PPN may still be able to provide 100% of a patient's nutritional needs if the formula volume is sufficiently high and the patient's weight is relatively low
- **Intradialytic parenteral nutrition (IDPN):** PN infused directly into the hemodialysis machine

Admixture

- An emulsion of lipid and the aqueous solution of dextrose, amino acids, electrolytes, and micronutrients:
  - 2:1 - the aqueous solution alone (dextrose and amino acid base)
  - 3:1 - dextrose, amino acid, and lipid base

Volume and water requirements

- 30-40 cc/kg/day
- Lower range as a person ages and has less lean mass and energy expenditure
- May be higher than above for persistent GI losses (eg, diarrhea, vomiting, ostomy, fistula, NG drainage)

Macronutrition ("base")

Nitrogen

- Source: Amino acids:
  - All essential amino acids
  - Many non-essential amino acids
  - Most do not contain taurine
- 4 kcal/g
- General requirements: 0.8-1.5 g/kg/day depending on metabolic needs and renal function
- Different proprietary preparations:
  - 10% solutions
  - 15% concentrated solutions for volume restriction
- <10% specialized solutions: containing taurine; enriched with branched chain amino acids
- Not all of the amino acid provided serves as protein substrate (need 1.0-1.8 g mixed amino acid/kg body weight to provide the equivalent of 0.8-1.5 formed proteins)

Carbohydrate

- Source: Dextrose (D-glucose)
- 3.4 kcal/g
- Typically 50% or 70% stock solution
- Requirements depend on energy expenditure (metabolic rate):
  - Minimum target: 100-130 g/day based on inhibition of gluconeogenesis
  - Glucose infusion rate range: 2-5 mg/kg/min
  - 60%-70% of nonprotein kcal (dextrose + lipid)
- Downtitrate with insulin resistance and hyperglycemia as needed

Lipid

- Soybean oil based (Intralipid) or combination of soybean and safflower oils (Liposyn II)
- Also contains eg, g phospholipids, glycerin
- 10 kcal/cc (9 kcal/cc lipid and 1 kcal/cc emulsifiers)
- 10 and 20% solutions may be infused alone
- 30% solution must be infused only as part of 3:1 admixture
- Contains essential fatty acids: linoleic acid (44%-62%; omega-6) and alpha-linolenic acid (4%-11%; omega-3) and other nonessential fatty acids
- Hypersensitivity reactions occur in <1%
- Targets:
  – 0.5-1 g/kg/day
  – 30%-40% nonprotein kcal (can be higher when using PPN)

Micronutrition

Electrolytes

Sodium:
- Necessary extracellular cation
- Major determinant of tonicity and osmolality
- Content range in PN is 0-154 mEq/L
- Available as Na-Cl, Na-acetate, and Na-phosphate
- Initialize based on:
  – Current serum Na
  – Current IV fluid used, or
  – IV fluid tonicity you would select:
    – Normal saline = 154 mEq/L sodium
    – ½ normal saline = 77 mEq/L sodium
- Adjust total Na content based on serum Na levels and volume status desired:
  – Can empirically decrease with heart, hepatic, or renal failure
  – Can empirically increase with volume contraction

Chloride:
- Anion that reflects acidity
- Available as Na-Cl or K-Cl
- Levels usually inversely related to bicarbonate
- May be elevated with renal tubular acidosis, GI bicarbonate losses (diarrhea), lactic acidosis, sepsis, etc.
- Patients with NGT drainage have increased requirements due to stomach losses

Electrolytes (cont.)

Potassium:
- Necessary intracellular cation
- May not be needed in patients with severe renal failure
- Content range in PN is 0-20 mEq/h (infusion time; if the PN infuses over 12 hours then the maximum K content is 240 mEq)
- Available as K-Cl, K-acetate, and K-phosphate
- If the K level becomes too high, then the PN bag will need to be aborted and then reformulated with lower K
- Unless patient has hyperkalemia at onset or severe renal failure, K should typically be included in all initial formulas
- Patients at risk for refeeding may have increased requirements early on due to rapid intracellular flux of potassium
- Patients with diarrhea may have increased requirements
- Patients on hydrocortisone infusions will typically have high requirements due to excess urinary losses

Acetate:
- Anion that reflects alkalinity
- Available as Na-acetate or K-acetate
- Add if acidosis present or expected
- Reflected by bicarbonate (total carbon dioxide levels) in lab tests
- May be elevated with volume contraction, steroids, GI proton losses [NGT output], renal tubular dysfunction, etc.
- Typically avoid in patients with liver disease (impaired utilization)

Calcium:
- Divalent cation
- Available as a calcium gluconate solution (4.7 mEq/gm)
- Usual amounts are 1.5-2 gm/day
- PN patients that may develop hypercalcemia are those receiving IV calcium boluses (ICU), with chronic immobilization and hyperresorption, or with primary hyperparathyroidism or humoral hypercalcemia of malignancy
- PN patients that may require larger amounts are those with intestinal malabsorption, vitamin D deficiency, or after head and neck surgery with iatrogenic hypoparathyroidism

Electrolytes (cont.)

Magnesium:
- Divalent cation
- Available as magnesium sulfate solution (8 mEq/gm)
- Usual amounts are 1.5-2 gm/day
- PN patients that may develop hypermagnesemia are those that are prerenal, s/p IV magnesium, or s/p cardiac surgery
- PN patients that may require larger amounts are those with intestinal malabsorption, diarrhea, s/p cis-platinum, or severely malnourished

Phosphate:
- Trivalent anion
- Available as Na-phos or K-phos; also present as phospholipid in the lipid emulsion and as potassium salt in amino acid solutions
- Usual amounts 10-15 mmol per 1000 kcal provided
- PN patients that may develop hyperphosphatemia are those with renal impairment and hypoparathyroidism
- PN patients that may require larger amounts are those at risk for refeeding syndrome or refeeding hypophosphatemia (severe/chronic malnutrition, alcoholism, anorexia nervosa, critical illness), insulinization, malnutrition, and vitamin D deficiency
- In general, hypophosphatemia at baseline is highly suggestive of vitamin D deficiency

Trace elements (required at <100 mg/day; "micronutrient")

- Necessary additives to prevent deficiency states with long-term PN use
- Reduce (1/2 amount) or omit MTE with frank hepatic insufficiency due to potentially toxic effects of copper and manganese (can re-add zinc 5 mg, selenium 60-100 mcg, and chromium 10-20 mcg as single entity products)

MTE-4

Zinc:
- 1 mg/cc (5 mg/cc in MTE-4 concentrate)
- Usual dose 2.5-5.0 mg
- Maximum dose up to 5-15 mg/day
- Can supplement individually with zinc sulfate, usually 5-10 mg
- Patient needs requiring increased zinc include chronic diarrhea, wound healing, critical illness
- Overtreatment can induce a copper deficiency

MTE-4 (cont.)

Copper:
- 4 mcg/cc (1 mg/cc in MTE-4 concentrate)
- Usual dose 0.3-5.0 mg
- Maximum dose up to 1 mg/day
- Can supplement individually with copper sulfate, usually 1 mg
- Overtreatment can induce hepatocellular toxicity

Manganese:
- 0.1 mg/cc (0.5 mg/cc in MTE-4 concentrate)
- Usual dose 60-100 mcg
- Maximum dose up to 0.5 mg
- Overtreatment can induce hepatobiliary toxicity and neurotoxicity

Chromium:
- 4 mcg/cc (10 mcg/cc in MTE-4 concentrate)
- Usual dose 10-15 mcg
- Maximum dose up to 100 mcg for up to about 14 days
- Can supplement individually with chromium chloride, usually 25-50 mcg
- Consider ↑ supplementation for severe insulin resistance

MTE-5 concentrate (MTE-4 + Se)

Selenium:
- 60 mcg/cc
- Usual dose 20-60 mcg
- Maximum dose up to 200 mcg/day
- Can supplement individually as selenious acid ("selenium") usually at 50-100 mcg/day
- Overtreatment associated with selenosis (GI symptoms, neurological Sx, cirrhosis, pulmonary edema, death)
- Consider ↑ supplementation for critical illness, catabolic illness

MTE-6 concentrate (MTE-5 + I)

Iodide:
- 75 mcg/cc
- Can supplement individually as sodium iodide 75 mcg
- Should omit with iodide allergy, concurrent amiodarone therapy

MTE-7 (MTE-6 + Mo)

- Molybdenum
- 25 mcg/cc
- Can supplement individually as ammonium molybdate
- Required for normal metabolism of sulfur amino acids

Ultratrace elements

(Constitute <1 mcg/gm of body; <0.0001% by weight) are not in PN.

- Tin
- Vanadium
- Cobalt (cobalt is provided as part of vitamin B12)
- Nickel
- Fluoride
- Arsenic
- Boron
- Bromine
- Cadmium
- Lead
- Lithium
- Silicon

Vitamins

(Essential organic micronutrients) as MVI - 13 (10 cc as dual vial [5 cc each] or two-chambered unit vial [requires mixing])

Vitamin A (retinol)	1 mg (3300 units)
Vitamin D (ergocalciferol)	5 mcg (200 units)
Vitamin E (di-alpha-tocopherol)	10 mg (10 units)
Vitamin K (phylloquinone)	150 mcg; may also dose as 0.5-1 mg/day or 5-10 mg/week
Vitamin B1 (thiamine)	6 mg; may supplement with 50-100 mg/day; loop diuretics and renal insufficiency associated with B1 (and other B-complex vitamin) depletion
Vitamin B2 (riboflavin)	3.6 mg
Vitamin B3 (niacin)	40 mg
Vitamin B5 (pantothenic acid)	15 mg
Vitamin B6 (pyridoxine)	6 mg; may supplement with 25 mg/day
Vitamin B7 (biotin)	60 mcg
Vitamin B9 (folic acid)	600 mcg; may supplement with 1 mg/day
Vitamin B12 (cobalamin)	5 mcg; may supplement with 25 mcg/day
Vitamin C (ascorbic acid)	200 mg; may supplement with 50-100 mg/day

Other additives

Nutrients

Carnitine:
- Dipeptide containing lysine and methionine
- Transports long-chain fatty acids from cytoplasm to mitochondria for oxidation
- Synthesis requires vitamin C:
  - Hepatic
  - Renal
- Features of deficiency states amenable to supplementation in PN:
  - Myopathy (eg, myalgia after hemodialysis)
  - Hepatopathy (eg, unexplained hyperbilirubinemia)
  - Dilated cardiomyopathy
  - Bone loss with home PN
  - Unexplained hypoglycemia
  - Unexplained hypertriglyceridemia
- Dosing: 0.5–2 g/day added to PN solution

Glutamine:
- Conditionally indispensible amino acid
- Formed from glutamic acid
- Gluconeogenesis precursor
- Immunomodulatory
- Trophic to intestinal mucosa
- Optimizes N retention
- Associated with improved ICU outcomes in some studies
- Enteral preparations are commercially available (0.3–0.57 g/kg/day)
- Parenteral preparations of glutamine or glutamine dipeptide are not commercially available in the U.S.
- Adverse effect: hyperammonemia

Supplemental C, B1, B6, folic acid, B12 (see above)

Supplemental Zn, Cu, Cr, Se, I (see above)

Drugs

Heparin:
Consider addition 1000 units per liter solution for hypercoagulable states to decrease risk of catheter thrombosis

Drugs (cont.)

Drugs not compatible in PN bag:
- Iron
- Steroids
- Octreotide

Insulin:
- Regular insulin
- Glycemic targets:
  - ICU: 80-110 mg/dL to 140-180 mg/dL depending on clinical setting and experience of ICU
  - Non-ICU: 100-140 mg/dL to 140-180 mg/dL depending on clinical setting and experience of glycemic targets
- Insulin strategies:
  - Strategy 1: provide 100% of the insulin requirement in the PN (start with 0.05-0.1 units per gm dextrose and titrate)
  - Strategy 2: provide nutritive insulin in PN (fixed dose of 0.05 - 0.1 units per gm dextrose) and add sq or IV insulin to correct to target
  - Strategy 3: no insulin in the PN and treat-to-target IV insulin (ICU setting)
- Transitioning PN insulin:
  - As patient tolerates more enteral nutrition, continue nutritive insulin in PN proportionate to the IV dextrose, synchronize sq insulin regimen where total daily dose is a fraction of the target insulin dose (about 60% IV insulin requirements or about 0.5 x kg lean dry weight)

H2-blockers
- Cimetidine: may have anti-neoplastic properties; more thrombocytopenia
- Ranitidine:
  - 150 mg/day usual dose
  - 75 mg/day with renal insufficiency
- Famotidine: most commonly used now
  - 40 mg/day usual dose
  - 20 mg/day reduced dose with renal insufficiency

Osmolarity of PN components

- Components:
  - Amino acid - 100 mOsmol per % final concentration
  - Dextrose - 50 mOsmol per % final concentration
  - Lipid - 1.7 mOsmol per g
  - Calcium - 1.4 mOsmol per mEq
  - Magnesium - 1 mOsmol per mEq
  - Potassium - 2 mOsmol per mEq
  - Sodium - 2 mOsmol per mEq
- Maximal mOsm/kg for 2:1 PPN = 800
- Maximal mOsm/kg for 3:1 PPN = 900
- No upper limit for central PN

Stability

Factors that destabilize lipid emulsion:

- Amino acid
- pH
- Dextrose concentration
- Electrolyte concentration
- Order of mixing in pharmacy

Calcium and phosphate stability:

- If Ca x Phos content is too high, then insoluble calcium phosphate precipitation occurs, which increases risk for pulmonary emboli
- Factors increasing Ca x Phos precipitation:
  - Amino acid (final concentration <2.5% and without cysteine)
  - pH >6.0
  - Temperature
  - Using calcium gluconate (instead of chloride salt)
  - Mixing calcium and phosphate in close sequence
  - Electrolyte concentration
  - Infusion after 24 hours of preparation
  - Calcium:Phosphate ratio <1:2
  - Total calcium and phosphate >45 mEq/L
  - Calcium:Phosphate solubility product >150

Stepwise PN formulation

- Assign total volume based on current IV fluid volume, computation (30-40 cc/kg/day), or judgment
- Build base formula that fits into total volume:

Stepwise PN formulation (cont.)	
Amino acid	Typically start with 1.0 gm/kg/day (no or mild stress) or 1.2 g/kg/day (moderate to severe stress) and up-titrate based on clinical setting and BUN to target 1.2 g/kg/day (no or mild stress) or 1.5 g/kg/day (moderate to severe stress) or 2.0 g/kg/day (profound protein losses due to extensive wounds, burns, diarrhea, or hemodialysis in the ICU)
Carbohydrate/dextrose	Start with 100-150 gm/day depending on glycemic status (lower dextrose with higher BG) and uptitrate once BG levels are controlled at or near glycemic target with insulin (see carbohydrate target and adverse effects below)
Lipid	Start without lipid, typically start 0.5 gm/kg/d and titrate up to 1.0 gm/kg/day. In ICU for the first 2-3 days and then slowly advance by 10-20 gm amounts to 0.5 gm/kg/day; ↓ or hold the lipid if the triglyceride levels are over 250 mg/dL (see lipid target and adverse effects below)

- Nonprotein (np; dextrose and lipid) targets and adverse effects:
  - Weight x target kcal/kg/day = total kcal needs per day:
    - ICU: 20 -25 kcal/kg/day
    - Non-ICU: 25 - 30 kcal/kg/day
    - Lower range with older age due to sarcopenia
    - Higher range with ↑ adiposity due to proportionately ↑ lean mass
  - Total caloric needs - kcal from amino acid (gm x 4 kcal/gm) = np kcal needs per day
  - 60%-70% np kcal = carbohydrate kcal/day; divide this by 3.4 kcal/gm to derive # gm dextrose per day
  - 30%-40% np kcal = lipid kcal/day; divide this by 10 kcal/gm to derive # gm lipid per day
- Base volume = gm amino acid divided by percent of the solution (6, 8.5, 10, or 15%) PLUS gm dextrose divided by 70% PLUS gm lipid divided percent of the solution (10, 20, or 30%); make sure the volume of the base is less than the total volume selected with about 100-150 cc leftover for electrolytes and other additives

Formulate electrolytes

Na (as phos + chloride + acetate):
- "Tonicity" of formula
- Initially match the tonicity of current IV fluid or what you would want it to be ("total Na"):
  - "Normal saline" = 154 mEq/L
  - "Half normal saline" = 77 mEq/L
  - "Quarter normal saline" = 38 mEq/L
- Then allot Na-phos amount from the total Na amount (usually 10-20 mEq/L):
  - 10 mEq Na-Phos = 7.5 mmol phos (3 cc solution)
- Then allot Na-Cl and Na-acetate amounts based on the patient's acid-base balance (usually no acetate initially unless frankly acidotic)

Potassium:
- Generally a little more than a routine maintenance IV fluid as "total K"; eg, about 30-40 mEq/L
- Then allot K-phos (usually 11-22 mEq/L):
  - 11 mEq K-Phos = 7.5 mmol phos (3 cc solution)
- Then allot K-Cl and K-acetate amounts based on the patient's acid-base balance (usual no acetate initially unless frankly acidotic)

Formulate other additives

Calcium	• 4.7 mEq/gm • Usually 1.5-2 g/day
Magnesium	• 8 mEq/gm • Usually 1.5-2 g/day
Multiple trace elements (MTE)	• Find out which brand/type the pharmacy has • Add standard amount (1 cc concentrate or 5 cc non-concentrate) • Reduce or omit with hepatic insufficiency or known toxicity
Multi-vitamin 13	10 cc standard

Consider adding to above
- Famotidine 40 mg (reduce or omit with renal insufficiency or low platelet count)
- Insulin 0.5-1 unit per gm dextrose (adjust based on glycemic targets desired)
- Carnitine 0.5-2 gm if patient at risk for deficiency state
- Heparin 1000 units/L if patient at risk for catheter thrombosis (very little evidence to support this)

- First 3 days: thiamine 100 mg and folic acid 1 mg, then reduce it to 50 mg and 0.5 mg, respectively, with ongoing catabolic illness or discontinue
- If at risk for deficiency: first 3 days - B12 25 mcg, C 100 mg, B6 25 mg and then reduce or discontinue
- If catabolic or in ICU: selenium 100 mcg
- If severely insulin resistant: chromium 25-200 mcg
- If diarrhea, catabolic, or has wounds: zinc 5-10 mg

Overfill

Pharmacy will routine overfill PN bag by 50 cc or more based on formula prescribed

Infusion schedule

- Order: "discontinue maintenance IV fluid when PN starts" so that the patient does not receive excessive IV fluids:
  - Exception: If patient on PCA pump (eg, postoperative analgesia) - "reduce maintenance IV fluid with PCA to KVO when PN starts"
  - Exception: If patient requires second IV for medicines and/or addition IV fluids as in ICU or recovery room - "reduce maintenance IV fluid per primary team orders when PN starts"
- Continuous infusion:
  - Divide total volume by 24 for infusion rate

Cycled Infusion

- Divide total volume by number of infusion hours minus one for "answer":
  - Half this "answer" is the infusion rate for first and last hour
  - The "answer" is the infusion rate for middle hours
  - Example: 2000 cc over 18 hours
  - Middle hours = 2000/17 = 117 cc/hour
  - First hour = 117/2 = 58 cc/hour
- Last hour = 58 cc/hour

Adjustment to protocol for PPN

Osmolality: Limit amino acid, dextrose, and sodium based on the total volume so that the mOsm/kg are <800 for 2:1 and <900 for 3:1

Adjustment to protocol for IDPN

To infuse over 3 hours only with HD, orders

- "IDPN to infuse over 3 hours with each HD session"
- "Dialysis team to write for IDPN on HD orders"
- Clarify in an advance with nursing and PN pharmacy to coordinate delivery of the IDPN in time for the HD and to deliver to the correct location (patient's hospital ward or the hospital dialysis center)
- Base formula is relatively standard:
  - Amino acid (15%): 80 gm
  - Dextrose: 150 gm
  - Lipid: 30 gm
  - No Na, K, Cl, acetate, Mg, Phos unless clearly needed
  - Calcium 1-2 gm
  - MTE routine
  - MVI routine
  - Insulin based on glucose determinations 2-3 hours into first IDPN infusion; can initialize with 0.5-1.0 unit/gm dextrose if patient has prior history of insulin requirement; adjust as needed
  - Carnitine 0.5-1 gm with ESRD; increase up to 2 gm if HD-related myalgias
  - Consider extra B-complex vitamins: thiamine 50-100 mg, folic acid 0.5-1 mg, B12 10-25 mcg, B6 10-25 mg

Other forms of renal replacement therapy

- Continuous Veno-Venous Hemofiltration (CVVH):
  - Concurrent infusion of central or peripheral PN without significant constraints on total volume as with IDPN: this is because CVVH typically has large replacement fluid infusion rates
  - No evidence that clinical outcomes are improved
- Peritoneal dialysis (PD):
  - Amino-acid containing PD solutions: 1%-1.1% amino acid instead of dextrose-containing bags; 1-2 bags per day titrated to a target total protein intake (about 1.2 g/kg/day)
  - Can ↑ AA levels and muscle AA uptake but no evidence that outcomes are improved
  - No evidence that clinical outcomes are improved

Supplemental parenteral nutrition (SPN)

Contemporary paradigm for nutrition support in critically ill patients

- Only 50%-60% of prescribed enteral kcal/day are actually delivered
- An accumulated energy and nitrogen debt adversely affects clinical outcome
- To supplement EN with a PN formula to prevent a critical (threshold effect) energy and nitrogen debt
- May be facilitated by providing as a 2:1 solution via non-dedicated central access or 3:1 solution via peripheral access

5.2.6   Complications

Refeeding

- Highest risk patients:
  - Severe malnutrition
  - Chronic malnutrition (but reported in patients without nutrition for as little as 48 hours)
  - Anorexia nervosa
  - Alcoholism
  - Neoplastic disease
- Related to the acute introduction of food (as carbohydrate) with intracellular phosphate trapping by hexokinase forming glucose-6-phosphate and further metabolism to ATP synthesis and lowering free intracellular phosphate
- This results in acute phosphate depletion as circulating phosphate rapidly enters cells down a concentration gradient
- Variable clinical picture
- Typically occurs 2-5 days after reintroduction of food (enteral or parenteral)
- Asymptomatic hypophosphatemia:
  - May or may not be associated with other features of refeeding syndrome
  - Treat by replacing phosphate enterally or parenterally

Symptomatic refeeding syndrome

- Hypophosphatemia is a consistent feature
- May be symptomatic related to:
  - Nutrient deficiencies
  - Tissue phosphate depletion: cardiac; neuromuscular
  - Rapid expansion of effective circulatory volume, heart failure, and respiratory failure, due to: IV fluid; IV sodium; carbohydrate stimulated insulin, which ↑ renal salt and water resorption; decompensated cardiomyopathy; respiratory insufficiency

- Also includes one of the following derangements:
  - Hypomagnesemia
  - Hypocalcemia
  - Hyponatremia
  - Hyperglycemia
  - Redistribution of micronutrients (vitamins and trace elements) creating deficiency states
- Prevent by avoiding rapid and high rates of carbohydrate, fluid, and sodium administration; and providing supplemental micronutrient support, especially B vitamins
- Treat by replacing acute deficiency states, managing acute cardiac and respiratory failure, and empirical lowering of nonprotein calories, volume, and sodium
- This is a potentially lethal condition mandating early and acute management

Overfeeding

- Principle that providing nutrition support (enteral or parenteral) in excess of metabolic needs creates a pathological condition with adverse clinical outcomes
- This is based on presumption that estimates of metabolic needs are accurate
- Carbohydrate overfeeding:
  - Hyperglycemia
  - Hepatopathy (steatosis)
  - Hypertriglyceridemia
  - Volume overload
- Fat overfeeding:
  - Hypertriglyceridemia
- Amino acid overfeeding:
  - Azotemia
  - Renal hyperfiltration (controversial)
  - Hyperammonemia (with concurrent hepatopathy or inborn error of metabolism)

Hyperglycemia

- Lack of incretin effect when no EN provided
- Prevent by limiting initial carbohydrate in patients with diabetes or at risk for hyperglycemia (eg, critical illness)
- Treat with insulin in PN (start with 0.1 unit/gm dextrose) and sq/IV insulin correction

Electrolytes

Parenteral nutrition associated liver disease[2]

- Ranges from mild elevations of transaminases (early) to steatosis, cirrhosis and end stage liver failure
- Steatosis:
  - Develops over weeks
  - Biopsy shows periportal lipid accumulation
  - Alkaline phosphatase levels rise first
- Steatonecrosis:
  - Develops over months
  - Biopsy shows panlobular fat and signs of liver necrosis
  - LFT's may not predict the course of disease
  - Reversible with cessation of TPN
- Cirrhosis:
  - Can occur after 20 months but usually after many years of TPN
  - May be as early as 6 months in patients with short bowel syndrome
  - Irreversible
- End stage liver failure:
  - Occurs in approximately 15% of patients who receive long-term parenteral nutrition

Possible PN related causes:

- Bacterial translocation (endotoxin)
- Overfeeding of carbohydrate
- Overfeeding of lipid (>1g/kg/day)
- Gallbladder stasis/biliary sludge
- Nutrient deficiencies: carnitine, glutamine, taurine, choline
- Amino acids (primarily infants)
- Soybean oil based lipid emulsions
  - Omega -6 fatty acids and phytosterols are associated with impaired biliary secretion
  - Downstream products of omega-6 fatty acids are proinflammatory

Management

Mild:

- First rule out non-PN related causes:
  - Preexisting liver disease, such as non-alcoholic fatty liver disease (NAFLD)
  - Medications
  - Metastatic disease involving liver
  - Systemic inflammation
  - Viral hepatitis
  - Sepsis
  - Reduce dextrose
  - Initiate small oral or enteral feeding if possible

Moderate:

- Reduce or discontinue MTE to avoid copper or manganese toxicity (and can re-add Cr, Se, Zn as single-nutrient products)
- Further reduce dextrose
- Reduce lipid
- Cycle PN infusion over 12-16 hours period instead of providing continuously over 24 hours/day
- Consider change AA solution to one that contains taurine (eg, Trophamine®)
- Consider add carnitine (1-3 g/day) to PN
- Consider oral glutamine (0.3-0.5 g/kg/day)
- Consider oral choline 3 g/d if patient can tolerate po
- Oral starchy food (source of trophic short-chain fatty acids)
- Consider prebiotics and probiotics
- Consider decontamination with antibiotics if biliary sepsis or bacterial overgrowth suspected (especially with short bowel syndrome)

End stage liver failure:

- Shunting and drainage procedures
- Intestinal rehabilitation
- Growth hormone
- Surgical elongation of intestinal mucosa
- Liver and small bowel transplantation

Future directions

Fish oil based lipid emulsions rich in omega 3 fatty acids rather may be hepatoprotective and used in the treatment of PN associated cholestasis. Not currently commercially available[56]

Metabolic bone disease

- Osteoporosis: Low bone mass and disruption of normal architecture of bone resulting in ↑ fragility
- Osteomalacia: Disorder of mineralization of newly formed matrix leading to soft bone, may have bone pain

Diagnosis

- DXA
- Osteomalacia: diagnosed by bone biopsy

Causes

- Metabolic acidosis:
  - Impairs vitamin D metabolism
  - Bacterial overgrowth (D-lactic acidosis)
  - Renal failure
  - Chronic diarrhea
- Negative calcium balance:
  - Inadequate provision of calcium or ↑ urinary losses
  - Cycled PN: ↑ urinary calcium losses
- Contamination of aluminum:
  - May be trace amounts in phosphate salts, calcium salts, ascorbic acid, heparin, MVI, trace elements, amino acids and magnesium
  - No longer a major problem
  - Impairs PTH secretion
  - ↓ 1,25 vitamin D
- Vitamin D deficiency:
  - Inadequate provision
  - Diarrhea
  - ↓ sunlight exposure
- Secondary hyperparathyroidism
- Vitamin K deficiency:
  - Leads to ↓ bone mineralization
  - Undercarboxylation of vitamin k dependent proteins (osteocalcin)
- Fluoride deficiency
- Medications:
  - Corticosteroids- reduce calcium absorption, ↑ hypercalciuria, cause hypogonadism
  - Methotrexate
  - Cyclosporine
  - Tacrolimus
  - Heparin

- Concomitant disease states:
  - IBD
  - Cancer
  - Amenorrhea
  - SBS

Management

- Calcium 15 mEq/day
- Phosphate 15 mmol/day
- Limit sodium: Causes hypercalciuria
- Reduce protein once nutritional status returns to normal (Not >1.5 g/kg/day):
  - Excess protein causes hypercalciuria
- MVI for adequate vitamin D and vitamin K
- Additional vitamin D as needed to maintain normal levels

Monitoring

- DXA
- Biochemical monitoring:
  - Collagen-crosslinks
  - Spot urine (N-telopeptide; NTx)
  - Serum (NTx or C-telopeptide; CTx)
  - Parathyroid hormone (PTH)
  - Bone-specific alkaline phosphatase
  - 25-OH vitamin D
  - 24 hours urine calcium
- Osteocalcin

Treatment

- IV bisphosphonate
  - Zoledronic acid 5 mg once every 1-2 years
  - Ibandronate 3 mg once every 3 months (if renal insufficiency)
  - Vitamin D levels should be >30 before treatment or patient should have
    received calcitriol for at least 2-4 weeks
- Teriparatide 20 mcg sq daily
- Can not use if uncorrected secondary hyperparathyroidism

Micronutrient disorders

- Deficiencies:
  - Zinc
  - Copper
  - Iron
  - Selenium
  - Chromium
  - Iodine
  - Vitamins A, D, E, K, C, B-complex
- Toxicities:
  - Aluminum
  - Vitamin A
  - Vitamin D
  - Manganese
  - Copper
  - Selenium
  - Chromium

Infectious: catheter related infections

Organisms in order of decreasing frequency

- Gram positive:
  - Coagulase negative Staphylococcus
  - Staphylococcus aureus
  - Enterococcus
- Candida species
- Gram negative bacilli:
  - Escherichia coli
  - Klebsiella
  - Enterobacter
  - Pseudomonas

Prevention

- Hand hygiene at time of insertion
- All inclusive catheter cart or kit
- Maximal sterile barrier precautions
- 2% chlorhexidine based antiseptic
- Subclavian vein preferred
- Avoid femoral vein if possible
- After insertion:
  - Disinfect catheter hubs and injection ports before accessing
  - Change dressings and perform site care with chlorhexidine based antiseptic every 5-7 days

Prevention (cont.)

- Antibiotic locks:
  - Filling the lumen of the catheter with a high concentration of antimicrobial solution and leaving the solution in place until catheter hub is reaccessed (ie, vancomycin, gentamicin, ciprofloxacin at 1-5 mg/mL mixed with 50-100 units heparin or saline in 2-5 mL volume)
  - Risks: toxicity, allergic reaction, bacterial resistance
  - May be used to salvage short term catheters colonized with coagulase negative staphylococcus or salvage of long term catheters with negative blood cultures and positive cultures from catheter 10-14 day for coagulase negative staphylococcus or gram negative bacilli

Management

- Draw at least one culture from central venous catheter and one culture by venipuncture
- Start with empiric coverage for gram positive, gram negative with plus or minus fungal and narrow after culture results
- If peripheral cultures negative and catheter removed, consider discontinue systemic therapy
- Empiric broad spectrum coverage eg,
  - Vancomycin or linezolid
  - Cefepime or carbapenem
  - Fluconazole or caspofungin

Short term catheters

- Coagulase negative Staphylococcus:
  - Remove catheter and treat with systemic antibiotics 5-7 days
  - If catheter retained, treat with systemic antibiotics and lock therapy for 10-14 days
- Staphylococcus aureus:
  - Remove catheter and treat with systemic antibiotics >14 days
- Enterococcus:
  - Remove catheter and treat with systemic antibiotics 7-14 days
- Gram negative bacilli:
  - Remove catheter and treat with systemic antibiotics 7-14 days
- Candida:
  - Remove catheter and treat with antifungals for 14 days after first negative culture

Long term catheters

- Coagulase negative Staphylococcus:
  - Retain catheter and treat with systemic antibiotics 10-14 days
  - Remove catheter if clinical deterioration or persistent bacteremia
- Staphylococcus aureus:
  - Remove catheter and treat with systemic antibiotic 4-6 weeks
- Enterococcus:
  - Retain catheter and treat with antibiotic lock therapy for 7-14 days
  - Remove catheter if clinically deteriorating or persistent bacteremia
- Gram negative bacilli:
  - Remove catheter and treat with systemic antibiotics for 7-14 days
  - Retain catheter and treat with antibiotic lock therapy for 10-14 days; if no response remove catheter and rule out complicated infection and if not present, treat for 10-14 days
- Candida:
  - Remove catheter and treat with antifungal for 14 days after first negative culture[55]

Hemostasis and thrombosis

- Bleeding at catheter site due to issues with initial placement or subsequent care
- Bleeding diathesis with underlying medical condition
- Higher rate of thrombosis with PICC: examine ipsilateral arm for edema and pain
- Hypercoagulable state with protein-wasting enteropathy
- Increased risks for thrombo-embolism with autoimmune disease, eg, scleroderma or malignancy, pancreatic cancer

Allergy

- Rare
- Avoid using IV lipid emulsions in patient with severe egg allergy
- Hypersensitivity reactions to lipids are prostaglandin mediated:
  - Symptoms: nausea, flushing, tachycardia, dyspnea, flushing, chest pain, back pain, headache, and sweats
  - Treat by discontinuing infusion
  - Antihistamines as needed
- Reported reactions to IV vitamins

Management

- Reverse-elimination protocol:
  - Start with 2:1 with only dextrose, amino acid, and minimal electrolytes
  - Stepwise addition of MVI, MTE, single-agent products and drugs
  - Then IV piggyback 10-20 g lipid over 5-10 hours with close observation (can stop without also stopping the 2:1 solution)
  - If tolerated, can slowly advance to targets
- If not tolerated, can try other products (eg, MVI), call allergy/immunology consultation, or steroid pretreatments

5.2.7 Monitoring

- Weight daily
- Daily input/output
- Biochemical (see table below)
- Clinical symptoms:
  - General well-being and energy
  - Hunger
  - Edema and puffiness
  - Pain with infusion
  - Shortness of breath with infusion
  - Body image
  - Urination and bowel movements

PN biochemical monitoring*			
Analyte(s)	Hospital (critically ill)	Hospital (noncritically ill)	Home
Na, K, Cl, CO_2, BUN, Cr	Daily	Daily until stable and then 3-4 times/week	1-2 times a week until stable and then weekly to biweekly
BG	Every 1-6 hrs depending on glycemic status and use of intensive insulin therapy	Daily until stable and then 3-4 times/week	1-2 times a week until stable and then weekly to biweekly
LFT	Daily to every other day	Daily to every other day until stable and then weekly	Weekly to biweekly

Analyte(s) (cont.)	Hospital (critically ill)	Hospital (noncritically ill)	Home
Mg, Ca, Phos	Daily to every other day	Daily until stable and then 2-3 times a week	Weekly to biweekly
TG	Daily until stable and then weekly	Daily until stable and then weekly	Weekly to biweekly
CBC	Daily	Daily until stable and then 2-3 times a week	Weekly to biweekly
PT (INR), PTT	Daily if anticoagulated or unstable otherwise, weekly	Daily if anticoagulated or unstable otherwise, weekly	Per routine if anticoagulated otherwise, weekly to biweekly
Vitamins A, D, E, K	Only if deficiency or toxicity suspected	Only if deficiency or toxicity suspected	Baseline and every 6 months
Se, Cr, Mn, Cu, Zn	Only if deficiency or toxicity suspected	Only if deficiency or toxicity suspected	Baseline and every 6 months
TSH PTH	N/A	N/A	Baseline and if clinically suspected
24 hours urine urea	After first 72 hours and then weekly to biweekly	After first 72 hours and then weekly to biweekly, if catabolic	Baseline and then q month to optimize N retention as needed
24 hr urine calcium, oxalate, citrate	N/A	N/A	Every 6-12 months

5.2.8   Trace element monitoring

Trace element monitoring in home TPN patients

- Patients receiving long term TPN require periodic monitoring of trace elements
- Consider testing selected trace element levels every 3-6 months
- Levels should be drawn when off TPN for at least four hours

Zinc	• Patients with intestinal losses (diarrhea or fistulas) may require increased supplementation • Serum levels may not reliably reflect status • Low alkaline phosphatase may be a sign of deficiency		
Copper	• May cause microcytic, normocytic, or macrocytic anemia • Monitor more frequently if patient has liver disease; may need to omit from TPN if cholestasis		
Selenium	• Should always be included in TPN • May have increase requirements with intestinal losses and stress • High MCV may be a sign of deficiency		
Manganese	• Toxicity is a common concern • Measure whole blood not plasma levels • Measure more frequently if patient has liver disease and manganese included in TPN; may need to eliminate MTE and add back individual components		
Chromium	• High glucose, high triglycerides may be signs of deficiency • Watch for signs of deficiency if excluded from TPN • Excessive loading may occur with renal failure		
Iron	• Common deficiency • Not provided in TPN • May need to supplement intravenously:		
	Iron sucrose (Venofer)	• Does not require test dose • Concentration 20 mg/mL (available in 2.5, 5, 10 mL vials) • Usual dosing 200 mg slow IVP over 2-5 min per day; repeat as needed • Risk of hypotension; low risk of anaphylaxis	
	Iron dextrose	• Prior to initiating IV iron dextran therapy, a one-time test dose of 25 mg (in adults) should be given IV • Anaphylactic type reactions typically occur within minutes; treat with epinephrine, diphenhydramine, steroids • Concentration 50 mg/mL • Usual dosing 100-200 mg (2-4 mL) iron diluted in 100 ml 0.9% saline or 5% dextrose solution over 30 min/day; repeat as needed	
	Iron dosing	• Total iron deficit [mg] = body weight [kg] x (target Hb-actual Hb) [g/dL] x 2.4* + depot iron [mg]	

5.2.9 Special considerations

Home TPN

Indications: prolonged PN therapy with significant intestinal impairment and severe malnutrition, or to support bowel rest as a primary therapy

Medicare reimbursability

- PN is considered reasonable and necessary for a patient with severe pathology of the alimentary tract which doesn't allow absorption of sufficient nutrients to maintain weight and strength commensurate with the patient's general condition
- Coverage of nutritional therapy as a Part B benefit is provided under the prosthetic device benefit provision
- The medical record, including the judgment of the attending physician must indicate that the impairment will be of long and indefinite duration (permanence)

Other logistics before committing to therapy – usually coordinated with hospital social worker

- Can patient manage home PN therapy
- If not, can patient be referred to a facility that can manage PN therapy
- Will third party payor reimburse
- Referral to a vendor (who then usually subcontracts with nursing agency)
- Suitable venous access device placed (PICC, indwelling catheter, port)

Formulation of home PN solution

- Cycle (usually over 10-12 hours)
- Should reach daily target volume, nonprotein kcal, nitrogen, and micronutrient needs

Other

- Monitor labs every 3-7 days at start until stable and then as infrequently as every 2-4 weeks depending on clinical status
- Pharmacists should routinely provide relevant "clinicals" on patients (overall status, volume status, amount or oral/enteral nutrition, planned medical procedures, other clinician orders) to assist with formula "rewrites"
- Pharmacy should be provided as much routine and emergency clinician contact information since reformulation is often performed over the phone
- Pharmacy will mail and/or fax clinical information to the clinician; orders will need to be signed promptly and faxed/mailed back to the pharmacist

- Clinicians should document all patient, pharmacy, and other management-related encounters; this is used to support clinician reimbursement for home PN oversight (billing details should be discussed with medical coder/biller professionals and/or the specific third party payor to optimize process)
- Every 6-12 months, a panel of biochemical tests should be ordered to screen for metabolic bone disease and micronutrient deficiencies/toxicities
- Nonspecific symptoms occurring within 1-2 hours of PN cycle start or finish can be managed by extending the usual ramps up or down from 1-2 hours (blunting the glycemic changes and/or lipid metabolism changes)

Red flags

"Red flags" that may require urgent/emergent care or referral to the emergency room include:
- Fever >101.5 °F
- (Nonspecific) acute decompensation
- Heart failure or acute fluid retention (not easily managed with an IV furosemide order)
- Altered mental status
- Psychological decompensation
- Complex electrolyte derangements
- Too many clinical problems to manage over the phone

Oley foundation

- National, independent, non-profit organization that enriches the lives of patients dependent on home PN and EN through education, outreach, and networking.
- The Foundation also serves as a resource for consumer's families, clinicians and industry representatives, and other interested parties.
- Programs are directed by the staff and guidance is provided by a board of dedicated professionals and patients.
- Contact information:
  - The Oley Foundation, 214 Hun Memorial, MC-28, Albany Medical Center, Albany, NY 12208-3478
  - www.oley.org
  - 1-800-776-OLEY - toll free in US and Canada
  - 1-518-262-5079 - calls from Europe and elsewhere
  - 1-518-262-5528 - fax

Effect on appetite

- Evidence not consistent
- Dextrose can stimulate or suppress
- Insulin-mediated (stimulates and suppresses)
- Lipids may have neutral or suppressing effects
- Amino acids (especially branched-chain) may stimulate
- Refeeding may generally stimulate
- Practical considerations:
  - If PN is suspected of suppressing appetite, can lower the lipid content first
  - When tapering off PN, lipid and carbohydrate should be lowered first, without changes in the amino acid content

Cyclosporine, hypocholesterolemia, and ulcerative colitis

- Cyclosporine binds to cholesterol
- Low cholesterol is associated with malnutrition
- Free cyclosporine levels can be abnormally elevated in patients with low cholesterol
- Excessive free cholesterol can bind to myelin and increase the risk for seizure
- Carbohydrate (not necessarily lipid) feeding with PN in malnourished ulcerative colitis patients not able to tolerate enteral nutrition can raise cholesterol levels and allow higher titrations of cyclosporine dosing
- As cyclosporine levels increase, this can also stimulate cholesterol synthesis so PN therapy is rarely needed for these purposes for more than a week
- Practical considerations: patients for cyclosporine treatment with cholesterol <80-100 range may benefit from a brief (5-7 day) course of PN to elevate cholesterol levels and allow full and earlier cyclosporine dosing

Discontinuing PN

- Reasons to consider aborting PN:
  - K >5 with K in bag
  - Phos >4.5 with phos in bag
  - Mg >2.5 with Mg in bag
  - BG >300-400 range (less extremes of hyperglycemia can be easily managed with insulin correction)
  - BG <80 with insulin in bag
  - Acute catheter-related infection
  - Destabilization of bag
  - Acute lipid-related symptoms, with lipid in bag
  - Acute catheter complications (bleeding, pain, thrombosis, etc.)
  - Certain procedures (PET scan [due to dextrose infusion], operative [at discretion of anesthesiologist], physical therapy [at discretion of physiatrist], etc.)

- There is no absolute need to infuse D10 or taper PN when discontinued, with following exceptions:
  - Patients may experience mild symptoms related to the down trend of BG or lipids and benefit from a one hour taper (half of the usual rate)
  - Patients with insulin in the bag may have less chance of hypoglycemia with a one hour taper (half of the usual rate)
- Patients on home PN or hospital cycled PN are routinely tapered up (at beginning of cycle for one hour at half the usual rate) and down (at end of cycle for one hour at half the usual rate)

5.3   Critical Illness

5.3.1   Metabolic mode

Platform to understand goals of nutrition and metabolic support in critically ill patient

Acute critical illness (ACI) – ICU day 0-2

- Initiated by stressor (injury, ischemia/infarction, infection, inflammation)
- Ventilator-dependent, in ICU, hemodynamic support
- Results in stress response: activation of the immune-neuroendocrine axis (INA); there is an evolutionary precedent ("Darwinian")
- Homeostasis: Feedback loops that maintain vital physiological functions in a narrow range (eg, pH and temperature); "resistance to change"

Acute critical illness (ACI) – ICU day 0-2 (cont.)

- Allostasis: Multiple physiological regulatory loops, involving brain function, that adjust homeostatic set-points for adaptation to stress states; "stability through change"
- Hormone (eg, insulin) resistance and hyperglycemia
- Hypermetabolism, catabolism, and cytokine-mediated substrate rerouting; ↑ (positive) acute-phase reactants (eg, C-reactive protein, complement, ferritin, plasminogen, ceruloplasmin); markers of inflammatory protein synthesis
- Depletion of negative acute-phase (or, reverse-phase) reactants (markers of structural protein synthesis)
  - Albumin (half life 20 days; large circulating pool)
  - Prealbumin (half life 2 days; small circulating pool; high ratio essential: nonessential amino acids; transthyretin)
  - Retinol-binding protein (half life 12 hours)
  - Antithrombin
  - Cortisol-binding globulin (transcortin)
- Abnormal body composition: anasarca primary due to fluid resuscitation

Therapeutic strategies

- Nutrition risk stratification: no validated score; NRS 2002 has been used in ICU nutrition studies
- Minimal interference with natural stress response
- Address overt nutritional deficiencies and metabolic derangements; consider early nutrition support if prolonged acute critical illness (below) likely to occur AND/OR patient at high nutritional risk
- Initiate tight glycemic control protocols with IV insulin:
  - Should be initiated at time of ICU admission
  - Use a validated dynamic, preferably nurse-driven, intensive IV insulin therapy protocol with documented safety and low rates of moderate (BG <70-80 mg/dL) and severe (BG <40 mg/dL) hypoglycemia
  - Consensus target is BG 140-180 mg/dL with ↓ glycemic variability
  - Lower targets (80-110 to 110-140 mg/dL) may be associated with improved outcomes in cardiac surgery patients provided they can be implemented safely (low rates of severe hypoglycemia as above)
  - Must be associated with protocols for transition to sq insulin and transfer from the ICU

Prolonged acute critical illness (PACI) - ICU day 3 or longer

- Failure of INA to down-regulate due to continued presence of stressors
- Altered neuroendocrine/hormonal function (eg, thyroid, adrenal, gonadal)
- Continued technological support and increased risk for morbidity and mortality
- No evolutionary precedent (no technology available for our hunter-gatherer ancestors)
- Allostatic load: Accrual of metabolic debt (eg, negative energy, protein, calcium status) due to sustained stress response
- Persistent insulin resistance, hyperglycemia, catabolism, and hypermetabolism
- Inadequate autophagy (inadequate removal of cellular debris: protein and mitochondria) leading to organ dysfunction
- Abnormal body composition
  - Depletion/catabolism of lean body mass (proteolysis of muscle to provide amino acids for gluconeogenesis and synthesis of acute phase reactants)
  - Depletion/catabolism of adipose tissue (lipolysis as fatty acid oxidation is increased)
  - Third spacing and anasarca (primarily due to hypoalbuminemia, which contributes to plasma oncotic pressure, and continued IV fluid load)
  - Typical appearance for adult kwashiorkor-like syndrome

Therapeutic strategies

- Continue tight glycemic control with IV insulin
- Initiate nutrition support protocols:
  - Timing of initiation can be based on nutritional risk
  - Target: 20–25 kcal/kg/day and 1.2–1.5 g/kg/day protein
    (Lower range for sarcopenia; Patients with obesity: 1.2 g/kg actual body weight
    or 2–2.5 g/kg ideal body weight; Use dry body weight (admission weight or usual
    weight) for patients with edema)
  - Enteral nutrition (EN)
  - Parenteral nutrition (PN; includes intradialytic PN [IDPN])
  - Combined modality (EN + PN)

Chronic critical illness (CCI) – ICU day 10–14 or longer

- Tracheostomy placed, indicating consensus opinion by ICU team that
  ventilator-dependence and critical illness will be prolonged further
- Allostatic overload: Metabolic debt at or near point that cannot be repaid
- CCI syndrome: Consistent clinical phenotype regardless of initial stressor(s)
  - Severe protein-energy malnutrition
  - Hyperglycemia
  - Bone hyper-resorption
  - Abnormal neuroendocrine function
  - Wounds
  - Elevated homocysteine (Hcy)
  - Critical illness polyneuropathy/myopathy
  - Depression and high symptom burden
  - High morbidity and mortality rates
  - Subtypes: **Type-1**: inflammation present &
    Type-2: no inflammation; prolonged mechanical ventilation due to
    severe neuromuscular impairment

Therapeutic strategies

- Tight glycemic control with subcutaneous insulin
- Continue PACI energy and protein targets (above)
- EN support with 24 hours continuous infusions of semi-elemental or
  specialized tube feeds
- PN support if unable to meet needs with EN, including tube feed interruptions
  >2–3 days
- Glutamine 15 g/day via enteral route (hold if hyperammonemic)
- Calcium 500–1000 mg elemental Ca^{++}/day (hold if hypercalcemic or
  hypercalciuric)

Therapeutic strategies (cont.)

- Vitamin D2 or D3 1000-2000 IU/day
- Calcitriol 0.25 mcg/day (hold if hypercalcemic, hypercalciuric, or hyperphosphatemic)
- Consider carnitine 0.5-1.0 g/day with severe cachexia, hepatic or renal insufficiency, valproate therapy, or unexplained hypoglycemia/hypertriglyceridemia/hyperammonemia
- Consider vitamin B12 1000 mcg sq q week + vitamin B6 25 mg/day + folic acid 1 mg/day for elevated homocysteine (Hcy); recheck levels in 2-4 weeks and down-titrate supplements
- Consider vitamin C 500 mg qd-BID + Zinc sulfate 220 mg/day + MVI 1 tab/day for wound healing; can taper after 2-4 weeks
- Adjuvant therapies:
  - Bisphosphonates: IV pamidronate 90 mg (or 1 mg/kg) x 1 dose provided vitamin D levels are replete (unless used for frank hypercalcemia)
  - Levothyroxine for confirmed hypothyroidism
  - Glucocorticoids
  - Physical therapy
  - Palliative care

Recovery from critical illness (RCI)

- Liberation from mechanical ventilation
- ↓ INA activation and inflammation
- Therapeutic strategies:
  - Continue tight glycemic control
  - Continue nutrition support: Increase target kcal to 25-30 kcal/kg/day; consider cycling EN infusions or transitioning to bolus EN; consider transition from nutrition support to oral (standard) nutrition as tolerated
  - Consider discontinuing nutritional supplements
- Intensify physical therapy and activity

5.3.2 Clinical evidence base

Monitoring

- Indirect calorimetry:
  - Underfeeding: Elevated measured energy expenditure (MEE) >> calories provided
  - Overfeeding: Suggested by elevated respiratory quotient or MEE lower than expected (and lower than calories provided); suggested by elevated total CO_2, elevated liver function tests, recalcitrant hyperglycemia, and azotemia (nitrogen overfeeding)
- Nitrogen balance studies: Generally inaccurate in the ICU due to ↑ urinary excretion of non-urea nitrogenous compounds and ↑ non-urinary nitrogenous losses (wounds, ventilator, stool); helpful if the urinary urea nitrogen is elevated
- Visceral proteins:
  - Albumin is nonspecific but sensitive marker of metabolic stress (inflammation) but not nutritional status
  - Prealbumin is nonspecific and poor marker of both metabolic stress and nutritional status due to confounding by renal/volume status
  - Both markers can indicate recovery

Therapeutic strategies

- Critical illness scoring systems:
  - Nutrition risk assessment based on status of body cell mass loss, severity of inflammation and expected clinical course, status of the GI tract, and risk of refeeding[57]
  - NRS 2002 based on weight loss history, body mass index, type of illness[58]
  - NUTRIC score based on conceptual model linking starvation, inflammation, nutrition, and clinical outcomes[59]

Nutrition support

- General consensus that EN should be provided by ICU day 2-3 depending on nutritional risk and titrated up to target quickly[60]
- North American paradigm is that PN does not need to be started in cases of insufficient EN until ICU day 8[61]
- European paradigm is mixed with some studies favoring early (ICU day 3) initiation of PN (alone or supplemental[62]) and others favoring late (ICU day 8) initiation of PN (alone or supplemental[63]); see ESPEN guidelines[64]
- Potential study confounders are
  - Trial design different from real-life management strategies
  - Appropriate comparator groups in PRCTs
  - Overfeeding and underfeeding when indirect calorimetry not used
  - Lack of sufficiently tight glycemic control or variability
  - EN and PN formulas not standardized

5.4 Nutritional Formulas

5.4.1 Standard formulas

Formula	Manufacturer	cal/can, Kcal/mL, Volume (mL), (%water)	Protein g/can	Fat g/can	Carb g/can	Fiber g/can	Protein source	Features patient type	Lactose-Free (L) Gluten-Free (G) Kosher (K), Halal (H)	Tube-feed (TF), Oral (O), Flavors
Compleat	Nestle	250 1.06 250 (85)	10	12	33	1.5	Chicken Milk	Formulated with real food for intolerance to semi-synthetic formulas	L G	TF unflavored
Jevity 1 cal	Abbott	250 1.06 237 (83)	10.4	8.2 20% MCT	36.5	3.4	Milk Soy	-	L G K H	TF unflavored
Nutren 1.0	Nestle	250 1.0 250 (84)	10	9.5 25% MCT	31.8	0	Milk	-	L G K	TF O Vanilla
Nutren 1.0 Fiber	Nestle	250 1.0 250 (84)	10	9.5 25% MCT	31.8	3.5	Milk	-	L G K	TF Vanilla
Osmolite 1 cal	Abbott	250 1.06 237 (84)	10.5	8.2 20% MCT	33.8	0	Milk Soy	-	L G K H	TF O unflavored

5.4.2   Concentrated standard formulas

Formula	Manufacturer	cal/can, Kcal/mL, Volume (mL), (%water)	Protein g/can	Fat g/can	Carb g/can	Fiber g/can	Protein source	Features patient type	Lactose-Free (L) Gluten-Free (G) Kosher (K), Halal (H)	Tube-feed (TF), Oral (O), Flavors
Iso-source 1.5 cal	Nestle	375 1.5 250 (81)	16.9	16.2	42	2	Soy	–	L G K	TF vanilla
Jevity 1.2 cal	Abbott	285 1.2 237 (80)	13.2	9.3 20% MCT	40.2	4.3	Milk Soy	Contains FOS	L G K H	TF O unfla-vored
Jevity 1.5	Abbott	355 1.5 237 (76)	15.1	11.8 20% MCT	51.1	5.3	Milk Soy	Contains FOS	L G K H	TF O unfla-vored
Nutren 1.5	Nestle	375 1.5 250 (78)	15	16.9 8.6g MCT/ can	42.3	0	Milk	–	L G K	TF O Vanilla
Nutren 2.0	Nestle	500 2.0 250 (70)	20	26 75% MCT	49	0	Milk	–	L G K	TF O Vanilla
Osmo-lite 1.2	Abbott	285 1.2 237 (82)	13.2	9.3 20% MCT	37.5	0	Milk Soy	–	L G K H	TF O unfla-vored
Osmo-lite 1.5	Abbott	355 1.5 237 (76)	14.9	11.6 20% MCT	48.2	0	Milk Soy	–	L G K H	TF O unfla-vored

5.4.3 High protein

Formula	Manufacturer	cal/can, Kcal/mL, Volume (mL), (%water)	Protein g/can	Fat g/can	Carb g/can	Fiber g/can	Protein source	Features patient type	Lactose-Free (L) Gluten-Free (G) Kosher (K), Halal (H)	Tube-feed (TF), Oral (O), Flavors
Fiber-source HN	Nestle	300 1.2 250 (81)	13.5	9.8 20% MCT	40	2.5	Soy	–	L G K	TF Unflavored
Iso-source HN	Nestle	300 1.2 250 (82)	13.4	9.8 20% MCT	40	0	Soy	–	L G K	TF unflavored
Promote	Abbott	237 1.0 237 (84)	14.8	6.2 23% MCT	30.8	0	Soy	Pressure ulcers	L G	TF O vanilla
Promote with Fiber	Abbott	237 1.0 237 (83)	14.8	6.7 23% MCT	32.8	3.4	Milk Soy	Pressure ulcers	L G	TF O vanilla
TwoCal HN	Abbott	475 2.0 237 (70)	19.9	21.5 23% MCT	51.8	1.2	Milk	Stress, volume restriction contains FOS	L G	TF O Vanilla, butter pecan
Peptamen Bariatric	Nestle	250 1.0 250 (84)	23.3	9.5	19.5	1.1	Milk	For critically ill obese patient	L G	TF unflavored

5.4.4 Liver disease

Formula	Manufacturer	cal/can, Kcal/mL, Volume (mL), (%water)	Protein g/can	Fat g/can	Carb g/can	Fiber g/can	Protein source	Features patient type	Lactose-Free (L) Gluten-Free (G) Kosher (K), Halal (H)	Tube-feed (TF), Oral (O), Flavors
Nutrihep	Nestle	375 1.5 250 (76)	10	5.3	72.5	0	Milk	Liver disease	L G K	TF Unflavored

5.4.5 Pulmonary

Formula	Manufacturer	cal/can, Kcal/mL, Volume (mL), (%water)	Protein g/can	Fat g/can	Carb g/can	Fiber g/can	Protein source	Features patient type	Lactose-Free (L) Gluten-Free (G) Kosher (K), Halal (H)	Tube-feed (TF), Oral (O), Flavors
Nutren Pulmonary	Nestle	375 1.5 250 (78)	23.7	17	25	0	Milk	Chronic respiratory disease Low carbohydrate	L G K	TF vanilla
Pulmocare	Abbott	355 1.5 237 (78)	14.8	22.1 20% MCT	25	0	Milk	COPD Low carbohydrate	L G K H	TF O vanilla

5.4.6 Diabetes

Formula	Manufacturer	cal/can, Kcal/mL, Volume (mL), (%water)	Protein g/can	Fat g/can	Carb g/can	Fiber g/can	Protein source	Features patient type	Lactose-Free (L) Gluten-Free (G) Kosher (K), Halal (H)	Tube-feed (TF), Oral (O), Flavors
Diabeti source AC	Nestle	250 1.0 250 (85)	9	7	33	0	Soy	Diabetes Contains real fruit and vegetables	L G K	TF Unflavored
Glucerna 1.0	Abbott	237 1.0 237 (85)	9.9	12.9 34.7% kcal as MUFA	22.8	3.4	Milk	Hyperglycemia	L G K H	TF O vanilla
Glucerna 1.2	Abbott	285 1.2 237 (81)	14.2	14.2 20% cal as MUFA	27.1	3.8	Milk	Hyperglycemia	L G K H	TF O vanilla
Glucerna 1.5	Abbott	356 1.5 237 (76)	19.6	17.8 29% cal as MUFA	31.5	3.8	Milk	Hyperglycemia	L G K H	TF O Vanilla
Nutren Glytrol	Nestle	250 1.0 250 (84)	11.9	11.3	25	3.8	Milk	Diabetes Contains prebiotics	L G K	TF O vanilla
Resource Diabetishield	Nestle	150 237	0	7	30	0	Milk	Diabetes Free free	L G K	O Mixed berry, Orange
Boost Glucose Control	Nestle	190 0.8 240	7	16	16	3	Milk arg	Diabetes	L G K	O Chocolate, vanilla

5.4.7   Renal

Formula	Manufacturer	cal/can, Kcal/mL, Volume (mL), (%water)	Protein g/can	Fat g/can	Carb g/can	Fiber g/can	Protein source	Features patient type	Lactose-Free (L) Gluten-Free (G) Kosher (K), Halal (H)	Tube-feed (TF), Oral (O), Flavors
Nepro with carb steady	Abbott	425 1.8 237 (73)	19.1	22.7	37.9	3.0	Milk	Stage V CKD hyperglycemia	L G	TF O Mixed berry, Vanilla Butter pecan
Nova-source Renal	Nestle	475 2.0 237 (71)	23.8	21.6	43.5	0	Milk	Renal failure	L G K	TF O Chocolate vanilla
Renalcal	Nestle	500 2.0 250 (70)	20.6	8.6	72.6	0	Milk	Acute renal failure For short term use Low protein Does not contain K, Na, Phos, fat soluble vitamins	L G K	TF unflavored
Suplena with carb steady	Abbott	425 1.8 237 (74)	10.6	22.7	46.5	3.0	Milk	Stage III and IV CKD hyperglycemia Low protein Low K, Phos, Ca, Na	L G	TF O vanilla

5.4.8 Immune enhancing/critical illness

Formula	Manufacturer	cal/can, Kcal/mL, Volume (mL), (%water)	Protein g/can	Fat g/can	Carb g/can	Fiber g/can	Protein source	Features patient type	Lactose-Free (L) Gluten-Free (G) Kosher (K), Halal (H)	Tube-feed (TF) Oral (O), Flavors
Pivot 1.5 cal	Abbott	355 1.5 237 (76)	22.2	12 20% MCT	40.9	1.8	Milk	Contains FOS, Arg, Gln Immunosuppressed pts, surgery, trauma, burn, head and neck cancer	L G H	TF
Impact	Nestle	250 1.0 250 (85)	14	6.9	32.9	0	Milk	Critical illness, surgery, high infection risk, contains arginine	L G K H	TF unflavored
Oxepa	Abbott	355 1.5 237 (78)	14.8	22.2 25% MCT	25	0	Milk	Critically ill SIRS or ARDS, vent Contains EPA and GLA	L G H	TF unflavored
Replete	Nestle	250 1.0 250 (84)	15.6	8.5 25% MCT	28.3	0	Milk	Wound management, surgery, burns, pressure ulcers	L G K	TF or oral vanilla
Replete fiber	Nestle	250 1.0 250 (83)	15.6	8.5 25% MCT	28.3	3.5	Milk	Wound management, surgery, burns, pressure ulcer	L G K	TF or oral vanilla

5.4.9   Elemental formulas

Formula	Manufacturer	Cal/can, Kcal/mL, Volume (mL), (%water)	Protein g/can	Fat g/can	Carb g/can	Fiber g/can	Protein source	Features patient type	Lactose-Free (L) Gluten-Free (G) Kosher (K), Halal (H)	Tube-feed (TF), Oral (O), Flavors
Peptamen	Nestle	250 1.0 250 (85)	10	9.8	31.8	0	Milk Peptide based Elemental	Impaired GI function	L G	TF or oral vanilla
Peptamen Junior	Nestle	250 1.0 250	7.5	9.6 62% MCT	34.4	0	milk	Peptide based, impaired GI function Ages 1-13	L G	TF or oral Vanilla, chocolate, strawberry
Peptamen AF	Nestle	300 1.2 250 (81)	18.9	13.7	26.7	1.3	Milk Peptide based Elemtental	Impaired GI function, high stress Contains fish oil	L G	TF Unflavored
Peptamen 1.5 with prebio	Nestle	375 1.5 250 (77)	17	14	46	1.63	Milk Peptide based	Impaired GI function Contains FOS	L G	TF Vanilla
Peptamen Junior 1.5	Nestle	375 1.5 250 (77)	17	14 60% MCT	46	0	Milk elemental	Peptide based, for ages 1-13, contains fish oil	L G	TF Unflavored

Elemental formulas (cont.)

Formula	Manufacturer	Cal/can, Kcal/mL, Volume (mL), (%water)	Protein g/can	Fat g/can	Carb g/can	Fiber g/can	Protein source	Features patient type	Lactose-Free (L) Gluten-Free (G) Kosher (K), Halal (H)	Tube-feed (TF), Oral (O), Flavors
Perative	Abbott	308 1.3 237 (79)	15.3	8.8 40% MCT	42.8	1.6	Milk Peptide based	Stress, pressure ulcers, fractures, wounds, burns surgery, contains arg and FOS	L G K H	TF Unflavored
Vital AF 1.2 cal	Abbott	237 1.2 284 (81)	17.8	12.8 45% MCT	26.2	1.2	Milk Peptide based elemental	GI dysfunction, inflammation Contains FOS	L G	TF O vanilla
Vital 1.0	Abbott	237 1.0 237 (84)	9.5	9.0 47.5% MCT	30.7	1.0	Milk Peptide based Elemental	GI dysfunction, inflammation Contains FOS	L G	TF O vanilla
Vital 1.5	Abbott	355 237 (76)	16	13.5 47.5% MCT	44.2	1.4	Milk Peptide based elemental	GI dysfunction, inflammation Contains FOS	L G	TF O vanilla
Vital HN powder	Abbott	300 1 packet (85)	12.5	3.35 45% MCT	55.4	0	Milk Peptide based elemental	GI dysfunction, inflammation Contains FOS	L G	TF O vanilla

Elemental formulas (cont.)

Formula	Manufacturer	Cal/can, Kcal/mL, Volume (mL), (%water)	Protein g/can	Fat g/can	Carb g/can	Fiber g/can	Protein source	Features patient type	Lactose-Free (L) Gluten-Free (G) Kosher (K), Halal (H)	Tube-feed (TF), Oral (O), Flavors
Vivonex plus (elemental powder)	Nestle	300 1 packet (83)	13.5	2	57	0	100% free amino acid	Severe GI dysfunction Contains gln, arg, BCAA	L G K	TF O
Vivonex RTF	Nestle	250 1.0 250 (85)	12.5	2.9 40% MCT	44	0	100% free amino acids	Severe GI dysfunction Stressed, low fat Contains gln and arg	L G K	TF O Un-fla-vored
Vivonex TEN (elemental powder)	Nestle	300 1 packet (83)	11.5	0.8	61.7	0	100% free amino acids	Severe GI dysfunc-tion Con-tains gln and arg	L G K	TF O

5.4.10 Oral nutritional supplements

Formula	Manufacturer	Cal/can, Kcal/mL, Volume (mL), (%water)	Protein g/can	Fat g/can	Carb g/can	Fiber g/can	Protein source	Features patient type	Lactose-Free (L) Gluten-Free (G) Kosher (K), Halal (H)	Tube-feed (TF), Oral (O), Flavors
Boost	Nestle	240 1.0	10	4	41	0	Milk Soy	Contains calcium 300 mg	L G K	O Vanilla, Chocolate, Strawberry
Boost plus	Nestle	360 1.5	14	14	45	0	Milk Soy	Contains prebiotics, high calcium 350 mg	L G K	O Vanilla, Chocolate, Strawberry
Ensure	Abbott	250 1.06 237	9	6	49	0	Milk Soy	-	L G K H	O Strawberry, vanilla, butter pecan, dark chocolate, milk chocolate, coffee latte
Ensure Plus	Abbott	350 1.5 237	13	11	50	0	Milk Soy	Contains prebiotics	L G K H	O Strawberry, vanilla, butter pecan, dark chocolate, milk chocolate, coffee latte

Oral nutritional supplements (cont.)

Formula	Manufacturer	Cal/can, Kcal/mL, Volume (mL), (%water)	Protein g/can	Fat g/can	Carb g/can	Fiber g/can	Protein source	Features patient type	Lactose-Free (L) Gluten-Free (G) Kosher (K), Halal (H)	Tube-feed (TF), Oral (O), Flavors
Ensure Enlive	Abbott	200 198	7	0	43	0	Milk	Fat-Free Supplemental not complete Multiple flavors (Apple, mixed berry)	L G	O
Impact advanced recovery	Nestle	340 237	18.1	9.2	44.7	3.3	Milk	Surgery	L G K H	O
Resource breeze	Nestle	250 337	9	0	54	0	Milk	Fat-Free Supplemental not complete Multiple flavors (orange, wild berry, peach)	L G K H	O

List of references

47 Sharma VK, Howden CW. Meta-analysis of randomized controlled trials of antibiotic prophylaxis before percutaneous endosciopic gastrostomy. Am J Gastroenteraol 2000;95:3133-3166

48 Latifi R: Nutritional therapy in critically ill and injured patients. Surg Clin North Am - 01-JUN-2011; 91(3): 579-93

49 Marik PE, Zaloga GP. Immunonutrition in critically ill patients: a systematic review and analysis of the literature. Intensive care med 2008;34(11):1980-90

50 Latifi R: Nutritional therapy in critically ill and injured patients. Surg Clin North Am - 01-JUN-2011; 91(3): 579-93

51 Marik PE, Zaloga GP. Immunonutrition in critically ill patients: a systematic review and analysis of the literature. Intensive care med 2008;34(11):1980-90

52 DeLegge MH: Enteral feeding. Curr ent opinion in gastroenterology 2008;24:184-189

53 Whelan et al. Mechanism, prevention and management of diarrhea in enteral nutrition. Current Opinion in Gastroenterology 27(2)2011 152-159

54 Enhanced protein-energy provision via the enteral route in critically ill patients: A single center feasibility trial of the PEP uP protocol Heyland DK, Cahill NE, Dhaliwal R, Wang M, Day AG, Alenzi A, Aris F, Muscedere J, Drover JW and McClave SA Critical Care 2010, 14:R78

55 Mermel LA, Alon M, Bouza E et al. Clinical practice guidelines for the diagnosis and management of intravascular catheter related infection 2009 infectious disease society of america . Clin Infect Dis 2009;49;1-45

56 Meijer VE, Gura K, Le HD, Meisel JA, Puder M: Fish Oil-Based Lipid Emulsions Prevent and Reverse Parenteral Nutrition-Associated Liver Disease: The Boston Experience. JPEN 2009;33:541-547.

57 Hiesmayr Curr Opin Clin Nutr Metab Care 2012; 15: 174-180

58 Kondrup et al. Clin Nutr 2003; 22: 321-36

59 Heyland et al. Crit Care 2011; 15: R268

60 Heyland et al. Crit Care 2010; 14: R78) to prevent underfeeding and critical energy debt (Reference: Villet et al. 2005; 24: 502-509

61 Cahill et al. JPEN 2011; 35: 160-168); see ASPEN guidelines (Reference: McClave et al. JPEN 2009; 33: 277-316

62 Heidegger et al. Lancet 2012; Dec 3 doi: 10.1016/S0140-6736(12)61351-8

63 Cesare et al. N Engl J Med 2011; 365: 506-517

64 Singer et al. Clin Nutr 2009; 28: 387-400

6 GI Disease and Post Surgery Abdomen

6.1 Gastrointestinal Disease

6.1.1 Irritable bowel syndrome

Chronic recurring and remitting functional GI tract disorder

Symptoms

- Episodic abdominal pain associated with alteration in bowel habits; bloating and flatulence are common
- May be constipation predominant, diarrhea predominant or mixed

Dietary management

- Avoid excess caffeine
- Moderate fat intake
- Probiotics:
  - Alteration of gut microbiota may be one of the etiologies of IBS
  - Small bowel bacterial overgrowth may contribute to symptoms
  - Postulated mechanisms of action of probiotics in IBS: Inhibition of pathogenic bacteria binding to the intestinal epithelial cells, enhancing barrier function of intestinal epithelial cells, acidification of the colon and suppression of the growth of pathogens
  - Most studied strains are Bifidobacterium and Lactobacilli
- Foods to eliminate for a 2 week therapeutic trial[65]:

– Dairy (lactose)	– Shellfish
– Wheat (gluten)	– Soybeans
– High-fructose corn syrup	– Beef
– Sorbitol	– Pork
– Eggs	– Lamb
– Nuts	

- Peppermint shown to be of benefit in some studies
- Guar gum may reduce symptoms

6.1.2 Gastroesophageal reflux disease (GERD)[66]

- Reflux of stomach contents causing troublesome symptoms and/or complications
- Transient relaxation of the lower esophageal sphincter (LES) occurs more often than normal
- May lead to metaplasia (Barrett's esophagus), dysplasia and adenocarcinoma

Dietary management

Avoid:

- Large or high fat meals 3 hours before bedtime
- Eating too fast
- High fat foods
- Spicy foods: irritate mucosa
- Chocolate
- Mint
- Citrus fruits
- Lying down after eating
- Specific beverages:
  - Alcohol: white wine and beer cause ↓ LES pressure
  - Caffeine
  - Coffee
  - Carbonated drinks: ↓ LES pressure

Other:

- Lose weight if obese
- ↑ dietary fiber

6.1.3 Crohn's disease[67]

- Croh'n disease (CD) is an idiopathic, chronic regional enteritis that most commonly affects the distal ileum but has the potential to affect any part of the gastrointestinal tract from mouth to anus.
- Transmural inflammation characterized by lymphoid hyperplasia, submucosal edema, ulcerative lesions, and fibrosis

Dietary management

- No role for PN as primary therapy:
  - PN may sometimes be needed to support patient through surgical or medical therapy
- No role for EN as primary therapy:
  - Primary EN is inferior to steroid treatment
- Bowel rest is not necessary (except with bowel obstruction, severe diarrhea, high output fistulas)
- No benefit to elemental diet as primary therapy:
  - Meta-analysis of 10 trials comparing elemental, semi-elemental and polymeric diet showed no difference in controlling exacerbations[68]
- Glutamine supplemented EN may be beneficial (unproven):
  - May lead to a reduction in intestinal damage
  - May improve of nitrogen balance
- Omega 3 fatty acids may help induce remission due to anti-inflammatory properties but results are inconsistent
- May be helpful to avoid high fiber foods during disease flares
- Terminal ileitis or prior terminal ileal resection increase risk for B12 deficiency

6.1.4   Ulcerative colitis

- Localized inflammation in the superficial layer of the colon mucosa
- Absorption of micronutrients is not impaired
- In ileostomy patients, bacterial fermentation of carbohydrate to short chain fatty acids is negligible, which might lead to loss of energy in the ileostomy fluid
- Pouches are colonized by a bacterial flora similar to colonic bacteria and fermentation occurs
- Probiotic preparations such as VSL#3 (containing bifidobacteria, lactobacilli and streptococcus thermophilus) may help maintain remission

6.1.5   Celiac disease

Immune mediated mucosal disease that involves the small intestine

- Gliadin peptides from gluten in diet result in an immunologic response
- Typical histopathological changes of celiac disease are flattened villi in the small intestinal
- Gluten-free diet should have good result
- Typical signs/symptoms include diarrhea, weight loss and malabsorption of nutrients

Micronutrient deficiencies

- Iron, folic acid, vitamin A and vitamin D are common and should be screened
- Deficiencies in vitamin B12, thiamine, and vitamin B6 are rare but may occur
- Deficiencies in selenium, copper, magnesium, and zinc have also been reported
- Calcium and/or vitamin D malabsorption and lead to secondary hyperparathyroidism and osteopenia, osteoporosis, or osteomalacia

Dietary management

- Must avoid wheat, barley, rye
- Oats can be a problem for some patients (cross-contamination)
- Typical gluten containing foods: Crackers, bread, cereal, cakes, cookies
- Hidden sources of gluten: Canned soups, salad dressings, ice cream, yogurt, pasta, processed meats, condiments, medications, lipsticks

6.1.6 Diverticular disease

- Diets high in red meat and low in fiber ↑ risk
- Consumption of nuts, corn or popcorn does not increase the risk of diverticulitis or diverticular bleeding
- There may be no basis for the long-standing recommendation that individuals with diverticulosis avoid high-residue foods
- Fiber deficiency may play a role in diverticular symptoms and complications
- Obesity, physical inactivity, smoking and alcohol are associated with increased risk

6.1.7 Acute pancreatitis[69]

- Extensive tissue damage due to the production of hydrolytic enzymes, toxins and cytokines may cause systemic activation of inflammation
- Characterized by hypermetabolism, hypercatabolism and negative nitrogen balance
- Unclear if pancreatic rest provides benefit
- Enteral nutrition is preferred when the GI tract is functional
- TPN may increase the risk of infection and the possibility of surgery when compared with EN[70]

Nutrition strategies[71]

Mild-moderate:

- NPO
- Advance to diet in 3-4 days
- Nutrition support usually not needed
- Start nutrition support if NPO >5-7 days

Severe:

- Early nutrition support is indicated:
  - EN
  - Generally preferred over PN
  - May be used in presence of fistulas, ascites and pseudocysts
  - Continuous EN preferred over bolus
  - Postpyloric placement is not usually required
  - Consider small peptide-based MCT oil formula
- PN:
  - Required in a minority of patients
  - Use when EN not tolerated or contraindicated
  - Fat emulsions are safe as long as baseline triglycerides <400 mg/dL
  - Control glucose
  - Consider glutamine (0.3 g/kg)
  - Avoid overfeeding
  - Protein 1.2-1.5 g/kg/day

6.2   Post Surgery Abdomen

6.2.1   Short bowel syndrome[72]

General

- **Definition**: Loss of absorptive capacity due to intestinal resection or GI disease
- Results in inability to maintain protein, energy, fluid, electrolyte, or micronutrient balance with normal diet
- **Causes**: postoperative resection, malignancy/irradiation, mesenteric vascular disease, Crohn's disease, trauma
- Normal small bowel length 365–600 cm; large bowel length 150 cm
- "Short bowel syndrome" generally occurs when there is less than 200 cm of intestine that is capable of nutrient absorption, together with GI fluid and electrolyte losses

TPN dependence

- >150–180 cm of small intestine does not usually require PN
- 60–90 cm small intestine plus intact colon usually needs PN <1 year
- <60 cm small intestine usually needs permanent PN

Pathophysiology

- Loss of intestinal absorptive surface
- More rapid intestinal transit
- Gastric hypersecretion inactivates pancreatic enzymes
- Retention of ileocecal valve lessens symptoms
- Loss of ileal tissue results in loss of "ileal brake" and speeds transit time
- Relative lactose intolerance occurs if there is resection of jejunum or proximal ileum, where lactase is synthesized
- Bile salts absorbed in distal ileum; loss leads to choleraic diarrhea and steatorrhea
- Lack of colon increases risk for greater fluid loss, faster gastric emptying (lack of peptide YY) and faster intestinal transit time also loss of calories through lack of metabolism of carbohydrate to short chain fatty acids

Clinical manifestations

- Diarrhea
- Steatorrhea
- Weight loss
- Vitamin deficiencies
- Trace element deficiencies
- Hyponatremia
- Hypokalemia
- Hypomagnesemia

Adaptation
- Process by which absorption improves
- Structural: ↑ absorptive area
- Functional: slower GI transit
- Histologic changes: ↑ in villus height, crypt depth, cell proliferation
- Can take up to 2 years after resection

Citrulline[73]
- Citrulline is a free amino produced by the metabolism of glutamine and proline in small bowel enterocytes
- The level of circulating plasma citrulline has been correlated with small bowel enterocyte mass and small bowel absorptive capacity
- Plasma citrulline of 15 may be a cut-off for the ability to wean from PN

PN management
See also parenteral nutrition support →130
- Protein 1-1.5 g/kg/day
- Total calories to 25-35 kcal/kg/day (lower if liver disease)
- Dextrose 2.5-5 g/kg/day (minimum 100-140 g); not to exceed rate of 5.5 mg/kg/min
- Lipids 0.5-1 g/kg/day

Enteral nutrition
- Can be considered if <2 L output per day
- If enteral feeding is needed then continuous feeds may be preferable at regular interval or bolus
- Initiate with elemental/semi-elemental feed; if tolerated, try to advance to intact protein feed

Dietary management
- Calories: 25-30 kcal/kg/day
- Protein: 1.0-1.5 g protein/kg/day
- Hypoosmolar feedings minimize GI fluid losses
- Generally small frequent meals 5-6 meals/day
- Glucose-electrolyte oral rehydration solution with sodium concentration of at least 70-90 mmol/L as needed
- Soluble fiber 5-10 g/day
- Intact colon:
  - Carbohydrates 50%-60%: complex carbohydrates, limit simple sugars, low lactose
  - Fat 20%-30%
  - Protein 20%-30% of total daily calories
  - Avoid oxalates

Dietary management

- No colon in continuity:
  - Carbohydrate 40%-50% of calories
  - Complex carbs
  - Limit simple sugars
  - Low lactose
  - Fat 30%-40%, LCT
  - Protein 20%-30%
  - Oxalate no restriction

Fiber supplements

Benefiber	2 teaspoons or 3 chewables or 3 caplets contains 3 g wheat dextrin
Citrucel	One scoop of powder contains 2 g of methylcellulose soluble fiber per dose; smart fiber caplets contain one gram per two caplet dose
Metamucil	One tablespoon powder contains 3 g fiber (2 g soluble fiber) psyllium, 6 capsules = 3 g fiber (2 g soluble fiber), 1 packet fiber singles = 3 g fiber (2 g soluble fiber)

Oral rehydration

- Oral rehydration solutions 1-3 L/day
- Intake must exceed ostomy output
- Keep urine sodium >20 mEq/L
- Keep urine output >1 L/day
- Can be administered via feeding tube
- Pedialyte powder packs, Pedialyte prepared solution and Pedialyte freezer pops. Provides per liter: Sodium 45 mEq ; Potassium 20 mEq ; Chloride 35 mEq; Zinc 7.8 mg; Dextrose 25 g; Calories 100
- Ceralyte 70 or 90 rice based oral rehydration drink 70 mEq/L and 90 mEq/L comes in ready-to-drink liquid form and packets to be mixed into water
- Home recipe for oral rehydration solution:
  - 1 liter water
  - 4 tablespoons sugar
  - ¾ teaspoon salt
  - ½ teaspoon baking soda or 1 teaspoon baking powder
  - ½ teaspoon 20% KCl powder
  - Sweetener/flavoring

Pharmacology	
Antidiarrheals	• Codeine 30-60 mg 1 hour before meals • Diphenoxylate (Lomotil) 2.5-5 mg 3-4 x per day take 1 hour before meals • Loperamide 2-4 mg 3-4x/day 1 hour before meals • DTO (tincture of opium 1%) 10-20 drops 1 hour before meals
Cholestyramine	Cholestyramine 2-4 g QID may help with unabsorbed bile salts

Antisecretory agents	• Control gastric hypersecretion (hypergastrinemia) which can exacerbate malabsorption and diarrhea
	• Necessary for first 6-12 months after resection
	• H2 blockers:
	  – Famotidine 40 mg BID
	  – Ranitidine 300 mg BID
	• Proton pump inhibitors:
	  – Omeprazole (Prilosec) 40 mg BID
	  – Pantoprazole(Protonix) 40 mg BID
	  – Lansoprazole (Prevacid) 30 mg BID
	  – Rabeprazole (Aciphex) 20 mg BID
	  – Esomeprazole (Nexium) 40 mg BID

Pancreatic enzymes	Pancreatic enzymes with meals may decrease diarrhea
Octreotide	Octreotide 50-200 mg tid can ↑ small intestinal transit time (not first line), may ↑ risk for cholelithiasis/cholestasis, hyperglycemia
Gattex™ (Teduglutide)[74]	See also Drug chapter →218
Zorbtive™ (somatropin rGH)	See also Drug chapter →218
Nutrestore™ (L-glutamine powder for oral solution)[75]	See also Drug chapter →218
A recent Cochrane review concluded that there are possible short term benefits in terms of weight gain or fat absorption but studies were small and "the available literature does not endorse the routine use of HGH or glutamine in short bowel syndrome."	

Supplements	
Calcium	• Typical dose: 1000–2000 mg/day • How supplied: – Calcium carbonate: 1250 mg = 500 mg elemental – Calcium citrate: 200, 315, or 600 mg tablets
Magnesium	• Typical dose: 50–500 mg/day • How supplied: – Mag tab SR (magnesium lactate) 840 mg (10% 84 mg elemental) – Slow mag (magnesium chloride) 535 mg (12%, 64 mg elemental) 71.5/119 mg – Magnesium gluconate 250 or 550 mg (8% elemental) – Magnesium oxide not recommended due to cathartic effects
Potassium	• Typical dose: 10–40 mEq • How supplied: – Potassium chloride 10 or 20 mEq tablet – 40 mEq/15 mL liquid
Zinc	• Zinc 50–150 mg/day elemental: – Zinc sulfate 220 mg = 50 elemental
Chromium	• Typical dose: 200–600 mcg/day • How supplied: 100, 200, 400 mcg tablet
Copper	• Copper 3–6 mg/day • How supplied: 3 mg tablets
Selenium	• Typical dose: 200–600 mcg/day • How supplied: 200 mcg tablets
Vitamin B12	• Vitamin B12 (if ileum resected need to supplement IM) • Typical dose: 1mg IM q 1–3 months • 1000 mcg tablets
Vitamin D	• Typical dose: 1000–4000 IU/day, 50,000 IU/week • How supplied: – Vitamin D3 400 IU, 1000 IU, 2000 IU – Ergocalciferol 50,000 IU capsule • Vitamin A: – Typical dose: 5000–10000 IU daily – How supplied: 5000, 10000, 25000 IU

Complications

- Electrolyte abnormalities: hyponatremia, hypokalemia, hypocalcemia, hypomagnesemia
- Catheter sepsis
- D-lactic acidosis[76]:
  - Colonic bacterial fermentation of unabsorbed nutrients, particularly simple sugars into D-enantiomer of lactic acid
  - Presents as altered mental status (MS), slurred speech ataxia (pt appears drunk)
  - Typically occurs after high carbohydrate feedings
  - Treatment: thiamine iv; enteral carbohydrate restriction; oral antibiotics-clindamycin 300 mg TID or vancomycin 125 mg QID or tetracycline 500 mg TID
  - PN induced liver disease
- Bacterial overgrowth presents with flatulence, bloating, crampy abdominal pain, foul smelling bowel movements, change in stool habits
  - Treatment
  - Cycled antibiotics
  - Rifaximin 1200 mg daily x 7-10 days
  - Flagyl 750 mg daily x 7-10 days
  - Non-lactobacillus based probiotics
- Cholelithiasis- due to absence of enteral intake:
  - Consider prophylactic cholecystectomy
  - Consider ursodiol prophylaxis
- Nephrolithiasis:
  - Usually calcium oxalate due to calcium binding to intraluminal fat leaves free oxalate in the lumen
  - Prevention
  - Low oxalate diet
  - Oral calcium supplements
  - High urine volume

Monitoring

- Vitamin D, vitamin A, vitamin E
- Selenium, iron, zinc, copper
- Essential fatty acids (triene:tetraene ratio)
- CBC, albumin, prealbumin, liver function, BUN, calcium, magnesium, phosphorus
- Urine output
- DXA
- Weight

Surgery[77]
Intestinal lengthening

Small bowel loop

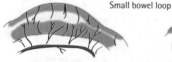 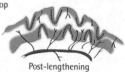

Pre-lengthening   Post-lengthening

- Bianchi procedure- involves dissection along the mesenteric edge of the bowel to longitudinal transection of the bowel to create two parallel limbs of smaller diameter then anastomosed together
- STEP serial transverse enteroplasty (preferred procedure):
  - Repeated application of a linear stapling device in zig zag fashion from opposite directions which partially divides the bowel
  - Since blood supply to the bowel comes from the mesenteric border of the bowel and traverses the bowel if all staple lines are kept perpendicular to the long axis of the bowel all segments of bowel remain well vascularized
  - Alternating the direction of the stapler from side to side creates a channel of bowel that is both smaller in diameter and longer in length than the original bowel

Intestinal transplant
- Usual indications:
  - Recurrent central line infection
  - Progressive liver disease
  - Progressive loss of central venous access; ie thrombosis of 2 or more central veins
  - Tumors

6.2.2   Chyle leak[78]

General

- Can be abdominal (triglycerides in paracentesis fluid) or thoracic (triglycerides in thoracocentesis fluid)
- Usually iatrogenic following surgery due to injury to the thoracic duct or other lymphatics
- Exacerbated by enteral nutrition (usually dietary long-chain fatty acids but in some patients with just clear liquids)

Nutritional and metabolic effects

- Fluid losses up to 2.5 L/day
- Metabolic acidosis
- Hyponatremia
- Hypocalcemia

- Depletion of body protein and fat:
  - Chylothorax leads to protein loss > chylous ascites
- Vitamin deficiency: Vitamins A, D, E, K
- ↑ metabolic demand

Nutrition management

- Conservative therapy can be tried for up to 2 weeks:

Output	Therapy
Low output <10 cc/day	Low fat diet
Moderate output 10-100 cc/day	Non-fat diet and MCT oil
High output 100-500 cc/day	Non-fat diet and MCT oil or NPO and PN
Very high output >500 cc/day	Surgical intervention

- Surgical intervention if:
  - Chyle leak >500 mL/day
  - Or in children >10 mL/kg/day
  - Or >100ml/day for each year of age for >5 days
  - Persistent leak >2 weeks
- Nutrition support should be started immediately
- Oral diet:
  - High protein
  - No long-chain fatty acids (<10 g/day): Requires transport from the gut through lacteal to thoracic duct
  - Medium chain triglycerides: Can substitute for long chain dietary fat; metabolized in the intestinal wall and transported directly into the portal circulation
  - When suspected leak resolved, advance to low fat diet
- Enteral feeding:
  - Elemental enteral formulas continuing less than 2%-3% total kcal as LCFA

Nutrition management (cont.)

- Risk of essential fatty acid deficiency if on a no fat diet >2 weeks
- Parental Nutrition:
  - Use when large chyle output or foregut reconstructive surgery
  - Consider also octreotide 100-200 mcg sq TID
- Monitor for deficiency of fat soluble vitamins, supplement vitamin D, maintain intravascular volume

6.2.3   Open abdomen[79, 80]

General

- Patients are hypermetabolic, high inflammatory response, high risk for malnutrition
- If full EN cannot be attained by 7-10 days then PN is indicated
- Patient have ↑ calorie and protein requirements:
  - Nonprotein calorie (25-35 kcal/day)
  - Protein 1.5-2.5 g protein/kg/day
- Wound granulation is sign of appropriate nutrition support
- UUN is erroneous due to unmeasured protein losses across open wound:
  - Estimated loss 2.9 g protein/dL of exudate
- Protein losses due to fistula are 1 g/500 mL fistula output
- Octreotide may decrease fistula output
- Acid blockers decrease volume of gastric secretions
- Length of bowel remaining should be documented

Management

- EN may be possible:
  - Early EN is associated with earlier fascial closure
- Follow albumin, prealbumin and CRP
- Enteroatmospheric fistula output should be estimated and replaced with electrolyte solution:
  - Foregut (esophagus, stomach): hypotonic
  - Midgut (duodenum, biliary tree, pancreas, small bowel): isotonic
  - Hindgut (colon, rectum): hypotonic

List of references

65 Wald a, rakel d: behavioral and complementary approaches for the treatment of irritable bowel syndrome. Nutr Clin Pract 23(3)284-292 2008.

66 vemulapalli, r: diet and lifestyle modifications in the management of gastroesophageal reflux disease, Nutr Clin Pract 23(3) 293-398 2008

67 Wiese DM, rivera r, seidner dl: is there a role for bowel rest in the nutrition management of crohns disease nutr clin parct 2008;23:309-317

68 Zachos M, Tondeur M, Griffiths AM. Enteral nutrition therapy for induction of remission in Crohn's disease. Cochrane Library 2007;2:1-36.

69 Mirtallo JM et al.: International Consensus Guidelines for Nutrition Therapy in Pancreatitis JPEN 36(3) 2012 284-291.

70 Marik PE, Zaloga GP. Meta-analysis of parenteral nutrition versus enteral nutrition in patients with acute pancreatitis. BMJ 2004; 328:1407.

71 Mirtallo JM et al. International Consensus Guidelines for Nutrition Therapy in Pancreatitis JPEN 2012;36:284-291.

72 Matarese LE. Nutrition and Fluid Optimization for Patients With Short Bowel Syndrome.JPEN J Parenter Enteral Nutr. 2012 Dec 21.

73 Bailly-Botuha C, Colomb V, Thioulouse E, Berthe MC, Garcette K, Dubern B, Goulet O, Couderc R, Girardet JP Plasma citrulline concentration reflects enterocyte mass in children with short bowel syndrome. Pediatr Res. 2009 May;65(5):559-63

74 Jeppesen PB, Pertkiewicz M, Messing B, Iyer K, Seidner DL, O'keefe SJ, Forbes A, Heinze H, Joelsson B. Teduglutide reduces need for parenteral support among patients with short bowel syndrome with intestinal failure.Gastroenterology. 2012 Dec;143(6):1473-1481.e3. doi: 10.1053/j.gastro.2012.09.007. Epub 2012 Sep 11.

75 Paul W Wales1,Ahmed Nasr2, Nicole de Silva3, Janet Yamada Human growth hormone and glutamine for patients with short bowel syndrome Cochrane Database Syst Rev. 2010 Jun 16;(6):CD006321

76 Peterson C D-lactic acidosis Nutr Clin Pract. 2005 Dec;20(6):634-45.

77 Thompson JS, Weseman R, Rochling FA, Mercer DA: Current management of the short bowel syndrome. Surg Clin N AM 91(2011)493-510.

78 Spain DA McClave SA Chylothorax and Chylous Ascites : ASPEN guidelines 2007

79 Friese RS: The open abdomen: definitions, management principles and nutrition support considerations. Nutr Clin Pract 2012;27:492-498)

80 Powell NJ and Collier B: nutrition and the open abdomen. Nutr clin pract 2012;29:499-506.

7 Metabolism

7.1 Determining Calorie Requirements

7.1.1 Definitions

Calorie	The amount of heat required to raise the temperature of 1 kg of water 1°C
Total energy expenditure (TEE)	Basal metabolic rate, thermogenic effect of food, and the effect of physical activity
Basal metabolic rate	Energy used by the chemical activities of resting tissue in a state of complete rest after a fast and at ambient temperature between 68–77°F (60%–75% TEE)
Thermogenic effect of food	The heat generated as food is digested
Physical activity	Activity in which work is performed and which increases metabolic rate
Resting energy expenditure (REE)	The basal amount of energy required for maintenance of lean functional body mass
Resting metabolic rate (RMR)	REE taken during a fast and allows for some movement (50%–70% TEE)
Calorimetry	Measurement of food energy in terms of kilocalories using a bomb calorimeter to burn the food and measure the heat energy produced
Direct calorimetry	Measurement of heat released from an individual at rest in a specialized chamber in which oxygen is introduced and expired CO_2 is measured
Indirect calorimetry	Indirect calorimetry measures the volume of oxygen consumed (VO_2) compared with the volume of carbon dioxide (VCO_2) expired
Metabolic cart	Device that measures oxygen consumed and CO_2 produced and then calculates the RMR for patients using the modified Weir equation

Modified Weir Equation	$RMR = [(3.9 \times VO_2) + (1.1 \times VCO_2) + (2.17 \times g \text{ of urinary nitrogen}] \times 1440$ or
	 Abbreviated $RMR = [(3.9 \times VO_2) + (1.1 \times VCO_2)] \times 1440$
	 • RQ: ratio of CO_2 produced to the volume of oxygen inspired (VCO_2/VO_2)
	 • RQ varies depending on fuel oxidized:
	   – RQ of 1.0 = compete oxidation of carbohydrate
	   – RQ of 0.7 = fat oxidation
	   – RQ of 0.85 = mixed diet
	 Handheld devices measure only VO_2 and RQ assumed to be 0.85

7.1.2 Determining REE with commonly used prediction equations

Harris Benedict[81] (REE) for healthy patients

- Men kcal/day = 66 +13.75 × body weight (kg) + 5 × height (cm) - 6.76 × age
- Women kcal/day = 655 +9.56 × body weight (kg) + 1.85 × height (cm) - 4.68 × age

Mifflin-StJeor[82] (REE) for healthy patients (includes obese patients)

- Men: 5 + 10 × actual body weight (kg) + 6.25 × height (cm) - 5 × age
- Women: 161 + 10 × actual body weight (kg) + 6.25 × height (cm) - 5 × age

Standard Penn State Equation for critically ill, ventilated patients[83]

RMR (kcal/day) = Mifflin (0.96) + Tmax (167) + Ve (31) - 6212

Modified Penn State Equation for critically ill, ventilated patients[83]

- RMR (kcal/day) = Mifflin (0.71) + Tmax (85) + Ve (64) - 3085
- Validated across BMI 21-49

Ireton-Jones Equations[84]: developed for hospitalized patients

- Ventilator-dependent: IJEE(v) = 1784 - 11(A) + 5(Wt) + 244(G) + 239(T) + 804(B)
- Spontaneously breathing: IJEE(s) = 629 - 11 (A) + 25 (W) - 609 (O)
- No additional factor is added for activity or injury

Faisy Equation (for mechanically ventilated patients)[85]

RMR (kcal/day): Wt (8) + Ht (14) + Ve (32) + Temp (94) - 4834

IJEE = kcal/day, A = age (yrs), Wt = actual wt(kg), G = gender (male=1, female=0), T = trauma, B = burn, O = obesity (if present=1, absent=0), v = ventilator, s = spontaneous, Ht = height, Temp = temperature (in °Celsius), Ve = expired minute ventilation in liters/minute, Tmax = maximum body temp in centigrade

7.1.3 Problems with prediction equations

- Variable metabolic response to critical illness:
  - 30%–50% are normometabolic
  - 15%–20% are hypometabolic
  - 35%–65% are hypermetabolic
- Obese patients have variable fat-free mass (metabolically active tissue)
- Most equations have not been validated in underweight patients
- Variable decline in metabolic rate with aging

7.1.4 Obese patients

- The higher the BMI, the less the relative contribution of lean body mass to total weight
- Using actual body weight can overestimate requirements because adipose tissue is less metabolically active than lean body mass
- Using ideal body weight will underestimate requirements because of increased
  metabolic activity of the extra lean body mass (20%–40% of excess weight)
- Indirect calorimetry preferred
- **Adjusted body weight:** Adjustment factor of 0.25 (actual body weight - ideal body weight) + ideal body weight
- **Hamwi's calculation to determine ideal body weight:**
  - **Men**: 106 + [height (inches) - 60 x 6]
  - **Women**: 100 + [height (inches) - 60 x 5]
- **Amato equation:** REE = 21 kcal/kg actual weight/day
- Hypocaloric (permissive) underfeeding[86, 87]: intentional administration of calories that are less than predicted energy expenditure
  - Target protein requirements are met
  - Rationale: positive nitrogen balance can be achieved at hypocaloric intake by increasing protein intake
  - May reduce complications of hyperglycemia, fluid overload, infection
  - Optimal calorie intake for obese patients in the ICU remains unclear: ASPEN guidelines[88] for critically ill obese patients: energy intake should not exceed 60%–70% of target energy requirements or 11–14 kcal/kg actual weight per day or 22–25 kcal/kg ideal body weight

7.1.5   Calorie requirement determination[89]

Calculated REE × activity factor = daily expenditure for healthy, non-pregnant patients for weight maintenance

Activity Factors for different levels of activity

- 1.2 sedentary activity
- 1.3 light activity
- 1.4-1.5 moderate activity
- 1.6-1.7 heavy physical activity

Daily calorie intake for healthy patients

- 25 kcal/kg for weight loss
- 30 kcal/kg for weight maintenance
- 35 kcal/kg for weight gain

Daily calorie intake for hospitalized patients

- Usual: 25-30 kcal/kg/day
- Burn patients: 35-40 kcal/kg/day
- Critically ill: 20-25 kcal/kg/day[90]
- American College of Chest Physicians
  - 25 kcal/kg actual or ideal body weight for stable patients
  - 27.5 kcal/kg for patients with SIRS

REE for hospitalized patients

- 100%-130% of REE for most patients
- 60%-70% REE for critically ill obese patients

7.1.6 Determining calories in partial and/or total loss of extremities[91]

The percent of body weight, for body parts removed with amputations, is important for calculating calorie needs

Relative weight of body parts (in amputation)

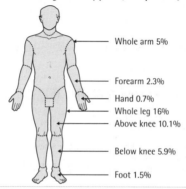

Whole arm 5%

Forearm 2.3%

Hand 0.7%

Whole leg 16%

Above knee 10.1%

Below knee 5.9%

Foot 1.5%

7.2 Nitrogen Balance

7.2.1 Definitions

- Simple: Nitrogen (N) input minus nitrogen output
- Positive Nitrogen balance is consistent with anabolism
- Negative Nitrogen balance is consistent with catabolism (illness or normal fasting)

Urinary urea nitrogen (UUN):

- Amount of urea excreted in the urine usually collected over 24 hours (normal range is 6-20 g/day)
- ↑ in diabetes, hyperthyroidism, increased dietary protein, and catabolic stress
- ↓ in liver disease, ↓ dietary protein, pregnancy, kidney disease, and drugs (furosemide, growth hormone, insulin, and testosterone)

- Urea is a metabolic end product of amino acid deamination or deamidation into carbon skeletons and ammonia:
  - Ammonia is converted into urea in the "urea cycle"
  - Ureagenesis reflects gluconeogenesis (certain amino acids are used as gluconeogenic substrates, namely alanine and glutamine)

Total urinary nitrogen (TUN)

- Amount of total nitrogen in urine
- Includes urea and non-urea nitrogen containing compounds (amino acids, ammonia, protein, and other)
- Can be measured directly (requires dedicated assay for TUN)
- Can be estimated as UUN/0.8 (underestimated during starvation and catabolic/critical illness)

7.2.2   Calculations

- Measure 24 hours UUN
- **Methods to compute Nitrogen (out):**
  - Method 1: Nitrogen (output) = UUN/0.8 + 2
    (the "2 g/day" estimates non-urinary nitrogen losses: expired, skin/wounds, GI/stool)
  - Method 2: Nitrogen (output) = UUN + 4
    (the "4 g/day" incorporates TUN and non-urinary nitrogen estimations together)
- **Determining Nitrogen (input):**
  - Review dietary records for protein intake
  - Divide daily protein intake by 6.25 ("6.25" = average ratio of weight of a specific amino acid to weight of nitrogen)
  - This number varies from amino acid to amino acid and from one protein source (eg, soy) to another (eg, whey)
- **Nitrogen balance = Nitrogen (input) − Nitrogen (output)**
- Example:
  - 24 hours UUN = 8.0 g
  - TUN = 10.0 g
  - Nitrogen (output) = 12.0 g (method 1 and 2 yield same result)
  - Dietary protein/day = 100.0 g
  - Nitrogen (input) = 100/6.25 = 16.0 g
  - Nitrogen balance = 16.0 − 12.0 = "+ 4.0 g/day" or "positive nitrogen balance"

7.2.3 Pitfalls

- Since nitrogen (output) increases with augmented dietary protein during periods of stress, the term "nitrogen balance" is supplanted with the term "optimizing nitrogen retention" since mathematically, the nitrogen (input) will rarely exceed the nitrogen (output)
- There are so many assumptions, estimations, measurement variances and flaws that the entire concept of nitrogen balance is usually not helpful. Specifically, a high UUN may imply minimal amounts of protein, whereas a low UUN lacks information.

List of references

81 Harris JA, Benedict FG. Biometric studies of basal metabolism in men. Washington, DC: Carnegie Institution of Washington, 1919
82 M D Mifflin, S T St Jeor, L A Hill, B J Scott, S A Daugherty, and Y O Koh: A new predictive equation for resting energy expenditure in healthy individuals. Am J Clin Nutr February 1990 vol. 51 no. 2 241-247
83 Swinamer DL, Grace MG, Hamilton SM, Jones RL, Roberts P, King EG. Predictive equation for assessing energy expenditure in mechanically ventilated critically ill patients. Crit Care Med 1990;18:657-61. Medline
84 Ireton-Jones C, Jones JD. Improved equations for predicting energy expenditure in patients: the Ireton-Jones equations. Nutr Clin Pract 2002;17:29-31. FREE Full Text
85 Faisy C, Guerot E, Diehl JL, Labrousse J, Fagon JY. Assessment of resting energy expenditure in mechanically ventilated patients. Am J Clin Nutr 2003;78:241-9. Abstract/FREE Full Text
86 Kushner RF and Drover JW: Current Strategies of Critical Care Assessment and Therapy of the Obese Patient (Hypocaloric Feeding): What Are We Doing and What Do We Need To Do: JPEN 35(1)2011 36S-43S.
87 Berger MM, Chioléro RL Hypocaloric feeding: pros and cons. Curr Opin Crit Care. 2007 Apr;13(2):180-6.
88 McClave SA, et al. Guidelines for the provision and assessment of nutrition support therapy in the adult critically ill patient: Society of Critical Care Medicine and American Society for Parenteral and Enteral Nutrition (A.S.P.E.N.). JPEN J Parenter Enteral Nutr. 2009; 33:277-316
89 McClave SA, Lowen CC, Kleber MJ, et al. Are patients fed appropriately according to their caloric requirements? JPEN J Parenter Enteral Nutr 1998; 22:375-381.
90 Frankenfield DC, Omert LA, Badellino MM, et al. Correlation between measured energy expenditure and clinically obtained variables in trauma and sepsis patients. JPEN J Parenter Enteral Nutr 1994;18:398-403. Abstract/FREE Full Text
91 Osterkamp LK: J Am Diet Assoc 1995;95:215-218.

8   Anorexia Nervosa

8.1   Diagnosis

Diagnostic guidelines (ICD 10)

Three components:
1) Restriction of energy intake
2) Fear of gaining weight
3) Disturbance in the way in which one's body weight or shape is experienced

For a definite diagnosis, all the following are required:

- Body weight is maintained at least 15% below that expected (either lost or never achieved), or Quetelet's body-mass index4 is 17.5 or less (4 Quetelet's body-mass index = weight (kg) to be used for age 16 or more. Prepubertal patients may show failure to make the expected weight gain during the period of growth).

- The weight loss is self-induced by avoidance of "fattening foods". One or more of the following may also be present: self-induced vomiting; self-induced purging; excessive exercise; use of appetite suppressants and/or diuretics.

- There is body-image distortion in the form of a specific psychopathology whereby a dread of fatness persists as an intrusive, overvalued idea and the patient imposes a low weight threshold on himself or herself

- A widespread endocrine disorder involving the hypothalamic-pituitary-gonadal axis is manifest in women as amenorrhea and in men as a loss of sexual interest and potency. There may also be elevated levels of growth hormone, raised levels of cortisol, changes in the peripheral metabolism of the thyroid hormone, and abnormalities of insulin secretion.

- If onset is prepubertal, the sequence of pubertal events is delayed or even arrested. With recovery, puberty is often completed normally, but the menarche is late.

8.2 Endocrine Abnormalities

- Hypogonadism: suppression of the hypothalamic-pituitary-gonadal axis results in low estrogen and low testosterone
- Bone loss:
  - Risk for osteopenia and osteoporosis
  - Bone loss is typically 2.5% per year
  - Young women may not achieve peak bone mass
- Hypercortisolemia
- Growth hormone resistance
- Part of female athlete triad (anorexia, osteoporosis, amenorrhea)
- Low T3 ("sick euthyroid")

8.3 Indications for Hospitalization

- Continued weight loss despite treatment
- Acute decrease in weight and food refusal
- Temperature <97 °F (36.1 °C)
- Systolic BP <90 mmHg
- HR <40 bpm at night <50 bpm during the day (risk of sudden death)
- Electrolyte abnormalities
- Hypoglycemia <40 mg/dL
- Cardiac arrhythmia
- Suicidal ideation
- Disturbance in consciousness

Indication for urgent hospitalization[92]

BMI of 13 kg/m^2 or lower may indicate a state of rapid physical deterioration and the approach of a life threatening stage.

8.4 Management

Multidisciplinary team: internist (cardiologist, endocrinologist as needed), psychiatrist, psychologist, dietitian

8.4.1   Refeeding[93]

- Initial 600-1000 kcal/day or 20-25 kcal/kg/day and 1.5-1.7 g protein/day
- Increase by 300-400 kcal/day every 3-4 days
- Never exceed 70-80 kcal/kg/day
- May need more than 3500 kcal to restore 1 pound of body weight due to increased thermic effect of food
- REE increases as feeding progresses
- Need to continually re-evaluate and monitor weights and adjust feeding regimen
- Goal: 0.2 kg/day weight gain or 2-3 pounds per week

8.4.2   Type of nutrition

- Oral feeding preferred
- Liquid nutritional supplements can be added to food
- TPN/EN indicated if:
  - Life threatening malnutrition (less than 40% IBW)
  - Noncompliance with treatment
  - Refusal to eat
  - Multiple previous treatment failures

8.5   Refeeding Syndrome

See also Refeeding→203

8.5.1   NICE guidelines for management of refeeding syndrome[94]

High risk of developing refeeding problems if:

One or more of the following:	OR	Two or more of the following:
BMI <16 kg/m^2		BMI <18.5 kg/m^2
Unintentional weight loss of >15% in the previous 3-6 months		Unintentional weight loss of >10% in the previous 3-6 months
Little or no nutritional intake for >10 days		Little or no nutritional intake for >5 days
Low levels of potassium, phosphorus, or magnesium before refeeding		History of alcohol abuse or drugs including insulin, chemotherapy, antacids, or diuretics

Prescription for the people at high risk of developing refeeding problems should consider[95]:

Check: K^+, Ca^{2+}, PO_4, Mg^{2+}

↓

Before feed start, administer Thiamine 200-300 mg daily orally and Vit B co strong1-2 table 3 times daily (Or full dose intravenous Vitamin B) and multivitamin//trace element supplement once daily

↓

Start feeding 10 Kcals/kg/day* Slowly increase feeding over 4-7 days

↓

Rehydrate carefully and supplement and/or correct K^+, PO_4, Ca^{2+}, Mg^{2+} levels: K^+ (2-4 mmol/kg/day), PO_4 (0.3-0.6 mmol/kg/day), Mg^{2+} (0.2 mmol/kg/day IV or 0.4 mmol/kg/day oral)

↓

Monitor K^+, PO_4, Ca^{2+} and Mg^{2+} for the first 2 weeks and act on as appropriate

* If severely malnourished, eg, BMI less than 14 kg/m^2 or negligible intake for 2 weeks or more, start feeding at maximum of 5 kcal/kg/day. Adapted from NICE and BAPEN guidelines

8.5.2   Management to avoid refeeding syndrome

- Start thiamine supplement 200-300 mg daily
- Provide multivitamin supplement
- Slowly increase feeding
- Monitor potassium, phosphorus, calcium, magnesium during first 2 weeks and supplement as needed

8.5.3   Laboratory abnormalities with refeeding syndrome

- Hypokalemia
- Hyponatremia
- Hypophosphatemia
- Hypocalcemia
- Hypomagnesemia
- Transaminitis
- Anemia
- Leukocytosis

8.6   Complications

- Fluid overload
- Cardiac failure
- Respiratory failure
- Hypoglycemia
- Gastrointestinal failure: slow gastric emptying, prolonged GI transit
- Wernicke's encephalopathy, Beriberi (thiamine deficiency)

List of references

92 Kawai K, Yamashita s, Yamanaka T, Gondo M, Morita C, Nozaki T, Takakura S, Hata T, Yamada Y, Matsubayashi S, Takii M, Kubo C, Sudo N. The longitudinal BMI pattern and body composition of patients with anorexia nervosa who require urgent hospitalization: A case control study Biopsychosoc Med. 2011; 5: 14.
93 Mehler PS, Winkelman AB, Andersen DM, Gaudiani JL. Nutritional Rehabilitation: Practical Guidelines for Refeeding the Anorectic Patient. J Nutr Metab. 2010; 2010: 625782.
94 NHS, Nutrition support in adults: Oral nutrition support, enteral tube feeding and parenteral nutrition, Clinical Guideline 32, Issue date: February 2006, pages 1-54, © National Institute for Health and Clinical Excellence.
95 Hisham Mehanna, Paul C Nankivell, Jamil Moledina, Jane Travis, Refeeding syndrome – awareness, prevention and management, Head Neck Oncol. 2009; 1: 4. Published online 2009 January 26. doi: 10.1186/1758-3284-1-4.

9 Cancer

9.1 Nutrition and Cancer Prevention

- High intake of nitrite cured foods (hot dogs, bacon) have been linked to cancers of the stomach, esophagus and pancreas
- Plant based diets are associated with a lower risk of cancer compared to diets high in saturated fat and meat
- Fiber, calcium, selenium and vitamin D are associated with anti-tumor properties related to colon cancer
- Highest preventative effect of diet for cancers of the stomach, esophagus, colon, mouth, throat and lung
- No single phytochemical accounts for protective effects
- Most studies found null associations between individual phytochemicals and cancer risk at various sites

9.2 Nutrition and Cancer Risk

- Obesity is associated with increased risk of cancers of the esophagus, pancreas, kidney, colon, rectum, breast (post-menopausal), endometrium, gall bladder and, non-Hodgkin's lymphoma
- SELECT trial (Selenium and Vitamin E Cancer Prevention Trial) studied oral supplementation with selenium (200 mcg/day) showed no protective effect of selenium and small increase in the risk of prostate cancer in men taking vitamin E alone[96]
- Beta carotene and lutein supplements associated with increased risk of lung cancer[97, 98]
- Alcohol intake is linked to risk of colon cancer

9.3 Malnutrition and Cancer

- Cancer cachexia: Progressive involuntary weight loss, tissue wasting, anorexia, muscle atrophy, hypoalbuminemia
- Causes:
  - Anorexia due to altered smell and perception of taste
  - Mechanical factors
  - Adverse effects of chemotherapy and radiation
  - ↑ pro-inflammatory cytokines
- May be present in early or late stages, predicts shorter survival

Malnutrition counseling algorithm[99]

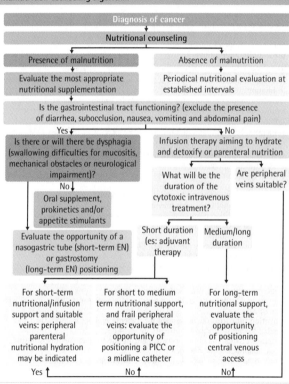

9.4   Nutrition Support in Cancer Cachexia

- Results in weight gain:
  - Increases fat mass than lean body mass
  - Progressive resistance training may augment lean body mass
- Improves nitrogen balance
- Does not improve albumin

Anti-cancer treatment

- Nutrition support should not be used routinely as adjunct to chemotherapy or irradiation
- Nutrition support is appropriate in patients receiving anticancer treatment who are unable to ingest or absorb oral nutrients for a prolonged period of time

Perioperative[100]

- Nutrition support is recommended for cancer patients who are moderately to severely malnourished or at risk of not receiving adequate nutrition orally for 7-14 days postoperatively
- Enteral Nutrition is preferred unless the GI tract cannot be accessed or is not functional
- Immune enhancing enteral formulas containing mixtures of arginine, nucleic acids and essential fatty acids may be beneficial
- Parenteral Nutrition is appropriate in malnourished patients who are anticipated to be unable to digest or absorb adequate nutrients enterally for more than 7-10 days
- It is appropriate to delay initiation of PN for up to 7 days if not clear needed
- Should typically be avoided if life expectancy is less than 40-60 days

Hematopoetic cell (bone marrow and stem cell) transplantation[101]

- All patients are at nutritional risk due to the underlying disease, treatment related toxicities and, graft versus host disease
- Mucositis, diarrhea, altered taste, anorexia, altered GI function may impair per oral intake
- Nutrition support is recommended for patients who are malnourished and unable to ingest or absorb nutrients for 7-14 days
- Enteral Nutrition may be especially difficult due to coagulopathy, sinusitis, ileus, abdominal pain, diarrhea
- Graft vs host disease (GVHD) generally results in poor oral intake and malabsorption, requiring nutrition support (usually PN)

9.5 Nutrition Assessment

SG-PGA (Patient generated subjective global assessment)[102]

- Designed for cancer patients
- Continuous scoring system
- Check-box format filled out by the patient plus physical examination
- Inquires about:
  - Weight change: 2 weeks, 6 months, 1 year
  - Symptoms of ↓ appetite, pain, nausea, diarrhea, vomiting, constipation, mouth sores, adverse smells, dry mouth and, funny taste or no taste
  - Food intake
  - Activities and function
- Given numerical score plus a rating of well-nourished, moderately malnourished/suspected malnutrition, or severely malnourished
- Score ≥9 indicates need for urgent nutritional intervention

9.6 Palliative Care

In the palliative care setting, nutrition support may be considered as part of compassionate care where net harm is acceptable:

- Medical futility but management of physical and emotional suffering requires nutrition support
- Patient must still allow blood draws at least once a week
- PN not expected to be associated with any increased risk of infection or biochemical derangement compared with a maintenance IV fluid that would be provided otherwise: eg, PN formula can be 5% dextrose with minimal amino acid and micronutrition
- Documented conversation that patient (or legal proxy) wants PN therapy in this setting (usually based on unsubstantiated fear that starvation will accelerate the dying process) and that the physician agrees with the decision
- If the physician does not agree with the use of PN and the patient (or proxy) continues to request it, then second opinions should be considered
- If/when the patient is discharged to a hospice setting, the hospice physicians general oversee the management of PN and may choose to discontinue it at the appropriate time
- Patients who have favorable benefit may be those with high performance status (Karnofsky score >50) inoperable bowel obstruction, minimal symptoms from diseases, indolent disease progression

References

96 Klein EA, Thompson IM Jr. Tangen CM et al. Vitamin E and the risk of prostate cancer: the Selenium and Vitamin E Cancer Prevention Trial. (SELECT)JAMA 2011:306(14):1549-56.

97 Omenn GS, Goodman GE, Thornquist MD, et al. Risk factors for lung cancer and for intervention effects in CARET, the Beta Carotene and Retinol Efficacy Trial. J Natl Cancer inst 1996;88:1550-59.

98 The effect of vitamin De and beta carotene on the incidence of lung cancer and other cancers in male smokers. The Alpha Tocopherol, Beta Carotene Cancer Prevention Study Group. N Engl J Med. 1994.330;1029-35.

99 Lidia Santarpia, Franco Contaldo, Fabrizio Pasanisi, Nutritional screening and early treatment of malnutrition in cancer patients, J Cachexia Sarcopenia Muscle. 2011 March; 2(1): 27–35. With permission.

100 Huhmann MB and August DA: Perioperative Nutrition Support in Cancer Patients. Nutr Clin Pract 27(5)2012:586-592.

101 August DA et al. ASPEN Clinical Guidelines: Nutrition Support Therapy During Adult Anticancer Treatment and in Hematopoietic Cell Transplantation. JPEN 33(5)2009; 472-500.

102 Bauer J et al. use of the scored patient generated subjective global assessment as a nutrition assessment tool in patients with cancer. Eur J Clin Nutr 2002 56(8)779-785)

10 Drugs

10.1 Appetite Stimulants

MA (oxandrolone): Anabolic steroid derivative of testosterone; **MA** (cyproheptadine): Serotonin and histamine antagonist with anticholinergic and sedative effects; indicated for treatment of allergies; **MA** (megestrol acetate): Progestin; **MA** (mirtazapine): norepinephrine antagonist and serotonin antagonist (norepinephrine, serotonin 5-HT2 and 5-HT3);
CI (oxandrolone): Prostate cancer, breast cancer, pregnancy, nephrosis, hypercalcemia;
CI (cyproheptadine): MAO therapy, angle-closure glaucoma, bladder neck obstruction, pyloroduodenal obstruction, symptomatic prostatic hypertrophy, stenosing peptic ulcer elderly debilitated patients, hypersensitivity; **CI** (mirtazapine): hypersensitivity to mirtazapine with MAO inhibitors;
AE (megestrol acetate): Nausea, diarrhea, impotence, rash, flatulence, hypertension, asthenia. Withdrawal can lead to adrenal insufficiency; **AE** (dronabinol): Abdominal pain, nausea, vomiting, dizziness, euphoria, (hallucination), paranoid reaction, somnolence, thinking abnormal; **AE** (mirtazapine): Somnolence, ↑ appetite, weight gain, dizziness, drowsiness, constipation, dry mouth, agranulocytosis (0,1%), Do not use with linezolid because of risk of serotonin syndrome, Warning: worsening suicide risk

Oxandrolone	PRC X, Lact-
Oxandrin *Tab 2.5 mg, 10 mg*	2.5 mg 10 mg daily Adults: 2.5 to 20 mg in divided doses given b.i.d. to q.i.d. for 2 to 4 wk; intermittent therapy repeated as prescribed. Maximum: 20 mg daily. Geriatric patients: 5 mg bid
Cyproheptadine	PRC B, Lact ?
Cyproheptadine HCL Tab *4 mg*	Available as 4 mg tablet Range 4-20 mg (2-3 times per day)
Megestrol acetate	EHL 13-104.9 h PRC X, Lact -
Megace ES *Tab 20 mg, 40 mg* *Oral suspension: 40 mg/mL or 125 mg/mL*	625 mg/5 mL **Appetite stimulation**: 800 mg/day of the regular megestrol suspension (40 mg/mL) or 625 mg/day of the ES formulation (125 mg/mL) **Breast cancer**: 40 mg four times daily

Dronabinol	EHL 19-36 h, PRC C, Lact ?
Marinol *Cap 2.5 mg, 5 mg, 10 mg* **Generic** *Cap 2.5 mg, 5 mg, 10 mg*	**Appetite stimulation:** Start with 2.5 mg PO twice daily before lunch and supper; reduce dose to 2.5 mg before bedtime if initial dose not tolerated; may increase dose to max 20 mg/day in divided doses, as needed/tolerated Chemotherapy induced nausea and vomiting: Start with 2.5 mg/m² PO 1-3 hours before treatment, then every 4-6 hours for total of 4-6 doses/day; escalate dose as needed by 2.5 mg/m² up to max 15 mg/m²

Mirtazapine	EHL 20-40 h, PRC C, Lact ?
Remeron *Tab 15 mg, 30 mg, 45 mg* **Remeron Soltab** *Tab (orally disint) 15 mg, 30 mg, 45 mg* **Generics** *Tab 7.5 mg, 15 mg, 30 mg, 45 mg; Tab (orally disint) 15 mg, 30 mg, 45 mg*	**Depression:** ini 15 mg/day PO, incr prn in intervals of >1-2 wk to 15-45 mg/day; DARF: see Prod Info

10.2 Prokinetic Agents

MA/EF (metoclopramide): inhibition of dopamine receptors ⇒ antiemetic; Stimulates motility of upper GI tract, sensitizes tissues to action of acetylcholine, antagonize central and peripheral dopamine rapid onset of action
AE (metoclopramide): dizziness, drowsiness, tiredness, head-ache, prolactin ↑, breast tenderness, gynecomastia, dry mouth, diarrhea, constip.; dyskinesias in CH, Parkinsonism;
CI (metoclopramide): pheochromocytoma, GI hemorrhage, obstruction or perforation, epilepsy, mental illness, Parkinson's disease; known hypersensit. to the drug, combination with MAO inhibitors, caution with children <14, and RF

Metoclopramide	EHL 2.5-5 h, Q0 0.7, PRC B, Lact ?
Reglan *Tab 5 mg, 10 mg,* *Tab (orally disint) 5 mg, 10 mgl, Inj 5 mg/mL* **Generics** *Tab 5 mg, 10 mg,* *Sol (oral) 5 mg/5 mL; Inj 5 mg/mL*	**GERD:** 10-15 mg PO qid; **postop nausea:** 10 mg IV/PO; **chemo-induced nausea:** 1-2 mg/kg/dose IV q2-4 h; DARF: GFR (mL/min) >50: 100%, 10-50: 75%, <10: 50%

10.3 Antifungal

MA (fluconazole): Inhibitor of fungal cytochrome p450 enzyme; **MA** (caspofungin): Treats Candidemia and invasive aspergillosis;
CI (fluconazole): Hypersensitivity, Caution with liver dysfunction, drugs that prolong QT interval; **CI** (caspofungin): hypersens. to caspofungin;
AE (fluconazole): nausea, abdom. pain, diarrhea, exanthema, headache, periph. neuropathy, LFT ↑, itching; **AE** (caspofungin): Diarrhea, fever, elevated liver function tests, hypokalemia, neutropenia, anemia, headache, phlebitis

Fluconazole	EHL 30 h, Q0 0.2, PRC D
Diflucan Tab 50 mg,100 mg, 150 mg, 200 mg, Susp 10 mg/35 mL; 40 mg/35 mL Inj 200 mg/100 mL, 400 mg/200 mL **Generics** Tab 50 mg,100 mg, 150 mg, 200 mg, Susp 10 mg/35 mL; 40 mg/35 mL Inj 200 mg/100 mL, 400 mg/200 mL	**Oropharyngeal/esophageal candidiasis**: first day 200 mg PO/IV qd, then 100 mg qd; **vaginal cand**: 150 mg PO as single dose; **systemic cand**: 400 mg PO/IV qd; **CH oropharyngeal/esophageal cand**: first day 6 mg/kg PO/IV qd, then 3 mg/kg qd; **systemic cand**: 6-12 mg/kg PO/IV qd DARF: GFR (mL/min) >50: 100%, <50: 50%

Caspofungin	EHL 9-11 h, PRC C, Lact ?
Cancidas Inj 50 mg/vial, 70 mg/vial	**Invasive aspergillosis:** d1 70 mg IV over 1 h, then 50 mg IV qd; DARF: not req

10.4 Antibiotics

MA (imipenem-cilastin): Active against gram positive and gram negative aerobes, and gram negative anaerobes, including Pseudomonas (ie. Enterococcus faecalis, Staphylococcus aureus (penicillinase-producing strains), Enterobacter species, Escherichia coli, Klebsiella species, Pseudomonas aeruginosa, Serratia species1, Bacteroides species including B. fragilis1); **MA** (cefepime): Active against gram positive (Staphylococcus aureus, streptococcus pyogenes, streptococcus pneumoniae, Streptococcus viridans) and gram negatives (Enterobacter, Escherichia coli, Proteus, Klebsiella species, Pseudomonas aeruginosa; **MA** (vancomycin): Effective against methicillin resistant staphylococcus aureus and used in patients who are penicillin allergic;
AE (imipenem-cilastin): N/V, diarrhea, liver enzymes ↑, allergic react, complete blood count changes, CNS DO; **AE** (cefepime): allergic skin reactions, Lyell-syndrome, anaphylaxis, N/V, diarrhea, transaminases↑, cholestasis, interstitial pneumonia, complete blood count changes, hemolytic anemia, creatinine↑, interstitial nephritis, superinfection by bacteria or yeasts; **AE** (vancomycin): allergic reactions, thrombophlebitis, ototoxicity, nephrotoxicity, complete blood count changes, red man/neck syndrome, N/V;

CI (imipenem-cilastin): CH < 3 mo, hypersens. to product ingredients, penicillins, cephalosporins, and other beta lactams; CI (cefepime): hypersensitivity to cephalosporins; CI (vancomycin): hypersensitivity to product ingredients

Imipenem + Cilastin	EHL 1 h, Q0 0.3/0.1, PRC C, Lact ?
Primaxin Inj 250 + 250 mg/vial, 500 + 500 mg/vial	**UTI, respiratory tract, intra-abdominal, gynecologic, bone/joint, skin infx, sepsis, endocarditis, polymicrobic:** >70 kg: 250–1000 mg IV q6, max 4 g/day, DARF: see Prod Info; Dose is reduced for renal impairment

Cefepime	EHL 2 h, PRC B, Lact ?
Maxipime Inj 500 mg/vial, 1 g/vial, 2 g/vial	**Severe UTI, intra-abdominal, skin infx:** 2 g IV q12 h; **pneumonia:** 1–2 g IV q12 h; **febrile neutropenia:** 2 g IV q8 h; DARF: GFR (mL/min): <10: 0.5–1 g q24 h, 11–30: 1–2 g q24 h; Requires dose reduction for renal impairment

Vancomycin	EHL 4–6 h, Q0 0.05, PRC C, Lact+serum-lev. (µg/mL): peak 30–40; trough 5–10
Vancocin HCL Cap 125 mg, 250 mg, Sol (oral) 250 mg/5 mL, 500 mg/6 mL, Inj 500 mg/vial Generics Inj 500 mg/vial, 1 g/vial, 5 g/vial, 10 g/vial, Inj 500 mg/100 mL, 750 mg/150 mL; 1 g/200 mL	**MRSA infx, other staphylococcal or streptococcal infx, endocarditis:** 1 g IV q12 h or 30 mg/kg/day IV div q12; **clostridium difficile diarrhea:** 125 mg PO qid for 7–10 d; DARF: GFR (mL/min): >50: 500 mg IV q12 h, 10–50: 500 mg IV q24–48 h, <10: 500 mg IV q48–96 h; Dose is reduced for renal dysfunction Infuse over 60 minutes; rapid infusion can cause hypotension

10.5 Antiobesity

MA/EF (orlistat): inhibition of gastric and pancreatic lipase $\Rightarrow$ hydrolysis of triglycerides into free fatty acids and monoglycerides $\downarrow \Rightarrow$ absorption $\downarrow$; **MA/EF** (phentermine): Norepinephrine releasing (amphetamine like) agent, anorexigenic effect $\Rightarrow$ loss of weight; **MA** (phentermine and topiramate extended-release): Phentermine is a sympathomimetic amine with pharmacologic activity. chronic weight management is likely mediated by release of catecholamines in the hypothalamus, resulting in reduced appetite and $\downarrow$food consumption, but other metabolic effects may also be involved; **MA** (lorcaserin): Lorcaserin is believed to $\downarrow$ food consumption and promote satiety by selectively activating 5-HT$_{2C}$ receptors on anorexigenic pro-opiomelanocortin neurons located in the hypothalamus; **MA** (alogliptin): slows the inactivation of incretin hormones GLP-1 (glucagon-like peptide-1) and GIP (glucose-dependent insulinotropic peptide);
AE (orlistat): Flatulence, bloating, abdominal pain, dyspepsia, diarrhea, resorption of fat soluble vitamin $\downarrow$. Vitamin supplementation at night is recommended; **AE** (phentermine): Agitation, insomnia, tachycardia, hypertension, headache, psychosis, nervousness, dizziness; **AE** (phentermine and topiramate extended-release): Paresthesia, Dry mouth, Constipation, URI , Metabolic acidosis, Nasopharyngitis, Headaches; **AE** (lorcaserin): Headaches, nausea, dizziness; **AE** (alogliptin): Nasopharyngitis (4.4%), headache (4.2%), and upper respiratory tract infection (4.2%);
CI (orlistat): Contraindicated in pregnancy, chronic malabsorption syndrome, cholestasis, may block levothyroxine absorption; must be dosed four hours apart; **CI** (phentermine): hypersensitivity to phentermine, hyperthyroidism, glaucoma, Contraindicated with MAO inhibitors, pregnancy, symptomatic CVS disease, advanced arteriosclerosis, mod-sev. HTN, pulmonary hypertension, history of drug abuse, alcoholism, agitated states, TCA. Use with caution in patient with high CAD risk; **CI** (phentermine and topiramate extended-release): Pregnancy, glaucoma, hyperthyroidism, MAO inhibitor therapy; **CI** (lorcaserin): Pregnancy; **CI** (alogliptin): History of a serious hypersensitivity reaction to alogliptin-containing products, such as anaphylaxis, angioedema or severe cutaneous adverse reactions

Orlistat	EHL 1-2 h, PRC B , Lact ?
Xenical *Cap 120 mg* **Alli** *Cap 60 mg*	**Obesity:** 120 mg PO tid with meals; Reduced dose: 60 mg TID marketed as Alli is available without a prescription DARF: not req Mean weight loss 2.59 kg at 6 months and 2.89 kg at 12 months 23, vitamin supplementation at night is recommended Fiber can reduce adverse effects

Phentermine	EHL 20 h, PRC C, Lact ?
Adipex-P *Tab 37.5 mg, Cap 37.5 mg* **Generics** *Tab 37.5 mg; Cap 15 mg, 30 mg, 37.5 mg*	**Obesity:** 8mg PO tid (30min ac) or 15-37.5mg PO qd; Can be used for up to 12 weeks; DARF: see Prod Info

Phentermine and topiramate extended-release	EHL 19-24 h, PRC X, Lact ?
Qsymia *Cap 3.75 mg/23 mg, 7.5 mg/46 mg, 11.25 mg/69 mg,15 mg/92 mg*	Qsymia 3.75 mg/23 mg (phentermine 3.75 mg/topiramate 23 mg extended-release) daily for 14 days; then increase to 7.5 mg/46 mg daily Do not exceed 7.5/46 mg with hepatic or renal impairment. Discontinue by taking a dose every other day for one week prior to stopping
Lorcaserin hydrochloride	PRC X, Lact ?
Belviq *Tab 10 mg*	Dose 10 mg BID; Discontinue if 5% weight loss is not achieved by week 12

10.6   Osteoporosis

MA (zoledronic acid): inhibitor of osteoclast-mediated bone resorption;
MA (ibandronate) andronate inhibits osteoclast activity and reduces bone resorption and turnover; **AE** (zoledronic acid): pyrexia, myalgia, headache, arthralgia, pain in extremity, flu-like illness, nausea, vomiting, diarrhea, eye inflammation; **AE** (alendronate): GI side effects, musculoskeletal; **AE** (risedronate): Back pain, arthralgia, abdominal pain, dyspepsia
AE (ibandronate): back pain, dyspepsia, pain in extremity, diarrhea, headache, and myalgia
AE (teriparatide): Arthralgia, pain, nausea; **AE** (denusomab): Musculoskeletal pain
CI (zoledronic acid): Hypocalcemia, pregnancy, CrCl <35 mL/min; **CI** (alendronate): In pregnancy; **CI** (risedronate): In pregnancy; **CI** (ibandronate): In pregnancy; **CI** (teriparatide): Prior irradiation involving the skeleton, bone metastases, skeletal malignancies, metabolic bone disease other than osteoporosis, hypercalcemic disorders, pregnancy;
CI (denusomab): Hypocalcemia, pregnancy

Zoledronic acid	PRC X, Lact -
Zoledronic Acid *Injection: 4 mg ; 4 mg/100 mL ; 5 mg/100 mL* *iv (infusion): eq 4 mg base/5 mL; eq 4 mg base/vial ; eq 5 mg base/100 mL* **Reclast** *Injection: 5 mg/100 mL* *iv (infusion): eq 5 mg base/100 mL*	**Osteoporosis:** 5 mg over 15 minutes iv every year **Osteopenia:** 5 mg over 15 minutes iv every 2 years

Alendronate	EHL up to 10 y, PRC C, Lact ?
Fosamax Tab 5 mg, 10 mg, 35 mg, 40 mg, 70 mg; Sol (oral) 70 mg/75 mL; **Generics** Tab 5 mg, 10 mg, 35 mg, 40 mg, 70 mg	**Postmenopausal osteoporosis PRO:** 5 mg PO qd or 35 mg qwk; **postmenopausal osteoporosis Tx:** 10 mg PO qd or 70 mg qwk; Must be taken 30 minutes before the first food or drink of the day with 6-8 oz water; do not lay down for 30 minutes; **steroid-induced osteoporosis Tx:** 5 mg PO qd (men and pre-menopausal women) or 10 mg PO qd (postmenopausal women not taking estrogen); **Paget's disease:** 40 mg PO qd for 6 mo; DARF: GFR (mL/min) 35-60: 100%, <35: not rec

Risedronate	EHL 1.5 h, PRC C, Lact ?
Actonel Tab 5 mg, 30 mg, 35 mg **Atelvia** Tab 35 mg	5 mg daily, 35 mg weekly, two 75 mg tablets per month or one 150 mg tablet per month Must be taken 30 minutes before the first food or drink of the day with 6-8 oz of water; do not lay down for 30 minutes after dose **Paget's disease:** 30 mg PO qd for 2 mo; **postmenopausal and steroid-induced osteoporosis:** 5 mg PO qd or 35 mg qwk; **osteoporosis in men:** 35 mg PO qwk; DARF: GFR (mL/min): >30: 100%, <30: not rec

Ibandronate	EHL 37-157 h, PRC C, Lact ?
Boniva Tab 2.5 mg, 150 mg, Inj 3 mg/3 mL	**Postmenopausal osteoporosis:** 2.5 mg PO qd or 150 mg qmo or 3 mg IV q3 mo; Must be taken with 6-8 oz of water; do not lay down for 60 minutes after dose; DARF GFR (mL/min) >30: 100%; <30: not rec

Teriparatide	EHL no data , PRC C, Lact -
Forteo Pen 600 mcg/2.4 mL	**Osteoporosis in postmenopausal women, primary or hypogonadal osteoporosis in men:** 20 mcg SC qd Supplied as multidose pen; self administered by patient. Maximum treatment duration is for 2 years

Denusomab	EHL 25.4 d, PRC X, Lact ?
Prolia *Vial 60 mg in a 1 mL solution*	60 mg every 6 months sq Supplied as prefilled syringe; administered by healthcare professional No dose adjustment necessary for renal impairment

10.7 Short Bowel Drugs

MA (teduglutide): Dipeptidyl-peptidase degradation-resistant GLP-2 analog, Enhances structural and functional integrity of the remaining intestine in SBS, promotes mucosal growth, inhibits gastric emptying and secretion, Reduced need for PN after 24 weeks treatment; **MA** (somatropin rGH): Stimulates structural and functional adaptation; **MA** (nutrestore): trophic to the intestine, enhances nutrient absorption;
AE (teduglutide): Abdominal pain, injection site reactions, nausea; **AE** (somatropin rGH): Common: peripheral edema (81%), Other: Associated with acute pancreatitis and impaired glucose tolerance; **AE** (nutrestore)
CI (teduglutide): cancer of the stomach, colon, liver, gallbladder, or pancreas;
CI (somatropin rGH): in active neoplasia, therapy should be carried out under the regular guidance of a physician who is experienced in the diagnosis and management of short bowel syndrome; **CI** (nutrestore): none

Teduglutide	EHL 1.3~2 h, PRC B, Lact ?
Gattex *5 mg/vial (as lyophilized powder) 3.8 mg/0.38 mL (after reconstitution)*	Dosing: 0.05 mg/kg once daily Injected subcutaneously in abdomen or thigh Requires prescriber training

Somatropin rGH	PRC B, Lact ?
Zorbtive *vial 8.8 mg*	0.1 mg/kg subcutaneously daily to a maximum of 8 mg daily Administration for more than 4 weeks has not been adequately studied Injected subcutaneously in the thigh or upper arm

Glutamine	PRC C, Lact ?
Nutrestore *5 g of L-glutamine powder*	Dosage 30 g daily in divided doses (5 g taken 6 times each day orally) for up to 16 weeks Each 5g dose should be reconstituted in 8-oz (250-mL) of water prior to consumption

10.8 GI Enzymes

MA/EF (pancrelipase): mixture of amylase, trypsin, and lipase;
AE (pancrelipase): skin rash, hypersensitivity, nausea/diarrhea with large doses, hyperuricemia, hyperuricosuria; **CI** (pancrelipase): hypersensit. to pork protein

Lactase	PRC N, Lact ?
Lactaid *Cap 3,000 FCC U, 9,000 FCC U* **Lac-Dose** *Tab 3,000 FCC U* **Lactose Intolerance, Lactrase** *Cap 250 mg standardized enzyme* **Generic** *3,000 FCC U*	**Lactose intolerance**: 1-2 capsules or tablets taken with milk or meals

Pancrelipase (lipase + protease + amylase)	PRC C, Lact ?
Creon *Cap DR 3,000 U + 9,500 U + 15,000 U; 6,000 U + 19,000 U + 30,000 U; 12,000 U + 38,000 U + 60,000 U; 24,000 U + 76,000 U + 120,000 U* **Pancrelipase** *Cap 5,000 U + 17,000 U + 27,000 U* **Pancreaze** *Cap DR 4,200 U + 10,000 U + 17,500 U; 10,500 U + 25,000 U + 43,750 U; 16,800 U + 40,000 U + 70,000 U; 21,000 U + 37,000 U + 61,000 U* **Ultresa** *Cap DR 13,800 U + 27,600 U + 27,600 U; 20,700 U + 41,400 U + 41,400 U; 23,000 U + 46,000 U + 46,000 U* **Viokace** *Tab 10,440 U + 39,150 U + 39,150 U; 20,880 U + 78,300 U + 78,300 U* **Zenpep** *Cap DR 3,000 U + 10,000 U + 16,000 U; 5,000 U + 17,000 U + 27,000 U; 10,000 U + 34,000 U + 55,000 U; 15,000 U + 51,000 U + 82,000 U; 20,000 U + 68,000 U + 109,000 U; 25,000 U + 85,000 U + 136,000 U*	**Pancreatic enzyme deficiency:** Start with 1,000 lipase units/kg of body weight per meal; increase as needed to max 2,500 units/kg of body weight per meal (or ≤ 10,000 lipase units/kg of body weight), or < 4,000 lipase units/g fat ingested per day

10.9　Ions, Minerals

10.9.1　Potassium

AE: N/V, belching, heartburn, flatulence, abdominal pain, diarrhea, mucosal ulcers, GI hemorrhage, ECG changes
CI: hyperkalemia, hyperchloremia, renal insufficiency, Addison's disease, acute dehydration, heat cramps

Potassium chloride　PRC C, Lact ?

Cena-k, Kaochlor, Kaon-Cl, Kay Ciel, K+ Care, K-Dur, K-Lor, Klor-Con, Klotrix, K-lyte, Micro-K, Rum-K, Slow-K Tab (ext.rel) 6.7 mEq, 8 mEq, 10 mEq, 20 mEq, 750 mg, 1500 mg, Tab (efferv) 20 mEq, 25 mEq, 50 mEq, Cap (ext.rel) 600 mg, 750 mg, Powder 15 mEq/pkt, 20 mEq/pkt, 25 mEq/pkt, Liquid 20 mEq/15 mL, 30 mEq/15 mL, 40 mEq/15 mL, 45 mEq/15 mL	**Hypokalemia Tx:** 40-100 mEq/day PO; 40-300 mEq/day IV, max 40 mEq/liter, max 15 mEq/h **hypokalemia PRO:** 20-40 mEq/day PO qd-bid

10.9.2　Calcium

AE (calcium IV): sensation of heat, fits of perspiration, BP ↓, N/V, arrhythmias
CI (calcium IV): hypercalcemia, nephrocalcinosis, digitalis intoxication, severe renal insuff.

Calcium acetate　PRC C, Lact ?

PhosLo Tab 667 mg, Cap 667 mg (169 mg Ca) **Generics** Tab 667 mg, Cap 667 mg, Inj 0.5 mEq/mL	**Hyperphosphatemia in end-stage RF:** ini 2 Tab PO tid with each meal, adjust dose based on serum phosphate; most patients require 3-4 Tab with each meal

Calcium carbonate　PRC C, Lact +

Alka-Mints Tab (chew) 340 mg **Calci-Chew** Tab (chew) 500 mg **Calci-Mix** Cap 500 mg **Caltrate** Tab 600 mg **Chooz** Tab (chew) 200 mg **Liqui-Cal** Cap 240 mg **Mallamint** Tab (chew) 168 mg **Nephro-Calci** Tab 600 mg **Os-Cal** Tab 500 mg, Tab (chew) 500 mg **Titralac** Tab (chew) 168 mg, 300 mg **Tums** Tab (chew) 200, 300, 400, 500 mg **Viactiv® Generics** Susp 500 mg/5 mL, Tab 260 mg, 500 mg, Tab (chew) 500 mg	**Hypocalcemia:** 1-2 g PO qd; **osteoporosis PRO:** 1-1.5 g PO qd; **RDA:** 1200 mg PO qd

Calcium chloride	PRC C, Lact ?
Generics *Inj 10% (10 mL) (1.36 mEq/mL)*	**Hypocalcemia**: 500-1000 mg IV q1-3 d; **magnesium intoxication**: 500 mg IV; **hyperkalemia**: dose must be titrated by ECG-changes

Calcium citrate	PRC C, Lact ?
Citracal *Tab 200 mg, Tab (efferv) 500 mg*	–

Calcium gluceptate	PRC C, Lact ?
Generics *Inj 22% (0.9mEq/mL)*	–

Calcium gluconate	PRC C, Lact ?
Generics *Tab 45 mg, 58.5 mg, 90 mg; Inj 10% Sol (0.46 mEq/mL)*	**Hypocalcemia**: 0.5-2 g slowly IV; 500-1000 mg PO bid-qid

10.9.3 Magnesium

AE: sleepiness, diarrhea, CNS disturbances, arrhythmias, muscle weakness, respiratory depression, flushing, hypotension; **CI:** restricted use in case of depressed renal function, 2 hrs preceding delivery, heart block; **IV:** AV block, myasthenia gravis

Magnesium gluconate	PRC A, Lact +
Magonate *Tab 500 mg (27 mg Mg), Liquid 54 mg Mg/5 mL*	**Hypomagnesemia**: 100-600 mg/day elemental magnesium PO div tid

Magnesium oxide	PRC A, Lact ?
Mag-Ox *Tab 400 mg [241.3 mg Mg (19.86 mEq)]* **Uro-Mag** *Cap 140 mg, [84.5 mg Mg (6.93 mEq)]* **Generics** *Cap 400 mg [84.5 mg Mg (6.93 mEq)], 420 mg*	**Hypomagnesemia**: 100-600 mg/day elemental magnesium PO div tid

Magnesium sulfate	PRC A, Lact +
Generics *Inj 80 mg/mL, 500 mg/mL, Inj 1g/ 100 mL, 2 g/100mL , 4 g/100 mL*	**Ventricular arrhythmias**: 1-6 g IV over several min, then 3-20 mg/min IV for 5-48 h; **preeclampsia, eclampsia**: 4 g IV, simultaneously 4-5 g IM each buttock; **preterm labor**: 4-6 g IV over 20 min, then 1-3 g/h IV

10.9.4 Fluoride

AE: N/V, diarrhea; **CI:** areas where water fluoride content is greater than 0.7 ppm

Fluoride	PRC no data currently available , Lact ?
Flura-Drops *Sol 5 mg/mL* **Flura-Tab** *Tab 1 mg* **Flura-Loz** *Tab (chew) 0.25 mg* **Fluoritab** *Sol 5 mg/mL,* *Tab (chew) 25 mg, 0.5 mg, 1 mg* **Luride** *Sol 0.5 mg/mL,* *Tab (chew) 0.25 mg, 0.5 mg, 1 mg* **Pediaflor** *Sol 0.5 mg/mL*	**Osteoporosis**: 25 mg PO bid (in combination with calcium citrate 400 mg bid)

10.9.5 Phosphorus

Phosphorus	PRC no data, Lact no data
K-Phos *Tab phosphorus/sodium/potassium 250 mg/298 mg/45 mg, Tab 500 mg (phosphorus/potassium 114 mg/144 mg)*	**Severe hypophosphatemia** (< 1 mg/dL): 1-3 g PO/PR

10.9.6 Iron

AE: N/V, diarrhea, constipation, dark-colored stools, when used intravenously: headaches, thrombophlebitis, allergic reactions, collapse
CI: hemochromatosis, hemolytic anemia, hemosiderosis, premature infants with vitamin E deficiency

Ferrous fumarate	PRC C, Lact +
Feostat *Susp 45 mg(15 mg iron)/0.6 mL, 100 mg (33 mg iron)/5 mL, Tab (chew) 100 mg (33 mg iron)* **Ircon** *Tab 200 mg (66 mg iron)* **Hemocyte** *324 mg (106 mg iron)* **Nephro-Fer** *Tab 350 mg (115 mg iron)* **Generics** *Tab 325 mg (107 mg iron)*	**Iron deficiency**: 2-3 mg/kg/day elemental iron PO div bid-tid

Ferrous gluconate	PRC C, Lact +
Fergon *Tab 240 mg (27 mg iron), 320 mg (37 mg iron)* **Generics** *Tab 300 mg (35 mg iron), 325 mg (38 mg iron)*	**Iron deficiency**: 2-3 mg/kg/day elemental iron PO div bid-tid

Ferrous polysaccharide	PRC C, Lact +
Ferrex *Cap 150 mg* **Fe-Tinic** *Cap 150 mg* **Hytinic** *Cap 150 mg* **Niferex** *Tab 50 mg, Cap 150 mg,* *Sol 100 mg/5 mL* **Nu-Iron** *Cap 150 mg, Sol 100 mg/5 mL*	**Iron deficiency**: 2-3 mg/kg/day elemental iron PO div bid-tid

Ferrous Sulfate	EHL 6 h, PRC C, Lact +
Feosol *Sol 220 mg(44 mg iron)/5 mL,* *Tab 325 mg (65 mg iron), 200 mg (65 mg iron), Caplet 45 mg iron/caplet* **Fer-Gen-Sol** *Sol 125 mg(25 mg iron)/mL,* **Fer-In-Sol** *Sol 90 mg(18 mg iron)/5 mL,* *125 mg (25 mg iron)/mL, Tab 325 mg (65 mg iron), Cap 190 mg (60 mg iron)* **Fero-Gradumet** *Tab 525 mg (105 mg iron)* **Mol-Iron** *Tab 195 mg (39 mg iron)* **Generics** *Sol 300 mg(60 mg iron)/5 mL,* *Cap (ext.rel) 150 mg (30 mg iron), 250 mg (50 mg iron), Tab 300 mg (60 mg iron), 325 mg (65 mg iron)*	**Iron deficiency:** 2-3 mg/kg/day elemental iron PO div bid-tid

Iron Dextran	PRC C, Lact +
DexFerrum *Inj 50 mg/mL* **InFed** *Inj 50 mg/mL* **Generics** *Inj 50 mg/mL*	**Iron deficiency anemia**: total dose (mL) = 0.0442 x (desired Hb – observed Hb) x kg + [0.26 x kg] IV

Iron Sucrose	EHL 6 h, PRC B, Lact +
Venofer *Inj 100 mg (iron)/5 mL*	**Iron deficiency anemia in chronic hemodialysis**: 100 mg IV 1-3x/wk up to a total of 1 g, rep prn

Sodium Ferric Gluconate	PRC B, Lact +
Ferrlecit *Inj 62.5 mg (iron)/5 mL*	**Iron deficiency anemia in chronic hemodialysis**: 10 mL (125 mg iron) diluted in 100 mL 0.9% NaCl IV over 1 h; rep. for a total of 8 dialysis sessions (1 g of iron)

10.10 Drugs Affecting Electrolyte Imbalances

10.10.1 Bisphosphonates

MA/EF: osteoclastic activity ↓ ⇒ osteal release of calcium ↓, bone degradation ↓;
AE: allergic skin reactions, hypocalcemia, GI DO; **AE (alendronate):** abdominal pain, musculoskeletal pain, headache, diarrhea, constipation; **AE (etidronate):** loss of taste, osteomalacia, GI complaints, bone pain; **AE (pamidronate):** myelosuppression, hypertension, thrombophlebitis, malaise, N/V; **AE (risedronate):** flu like syndrome, diarrhea, arthralgia, headache, abdominal pain, rash; **AE (tiludronate):** N/V/diarrhea, skin reactions, edema, chest pain;
CI: renal insuffiency, acute GI inflammation, CH; **CI (alendronate):** hypersensitivity to alendronate products, hypocalcemia, esophageal DO, inability to stand or sit upright for 30min, CrCl <35mL/min; **CI (clodranate):** Cr>440 umol/L, severe inflammation of GI tract; **CI (etidronate):** hypersensitivity to etidronate products, osteomalacia; **CI (pamidronate):** hypersensitivity to bisphosphonates; **CI (risedronate):** hypocalcemia, hypersensitivity to risedronate products; **CI (tiludronate):** hypersensitivity to tiludronate products

Alendronate	EHL up to 10 y, PRC C, Lact
Fosamax Tab 5 mg, 10 mg, 35 mg, 40 mg, 70 mg; Sol (oral) 70 mg/75 mL; **Generics** Tab 5 mg, 10 mg, 35 mg, 40 mg, 70 mg	**Postmenopausal osteoporosis PRO:** 5 mg PO qd or 35 mg qwk; **postmenopausal osteoporosis Tx:** 10 mg PO qd or 70 mg qwk; **steroid-induced osteoporosis Tx:** 5 mg PO qd (men and pre-menopausal women) or 10 mg PO qd (postmenopausal women not taking estrogen); **Paget's disease:** 40 mg PO qd for 6 mo; DARF: GFR (mL/min) 35-60: 100%, <35: not rec

Etidronate	EHL 1-6 h (or); 5.3-6.7h (IV), PRC C, Lact
Didronel Tab 200 mg, 400 mg, **Generics** Tab 200 mg, 400 mg	**Paget's disease:** 5-10 mg/kg/day PO for 6 mo or 11-20 mg/kg/day PO for 3 mo **heterotopic ossification with hip replacement:** 20 mg/kg/day PO 1 mo before and 3 mo after surgery; **heterotopic ossification with spinal cord injury:** 20 mg, kg/day PO for 2 wk, then 10 mg/kg/day PO for 10 wk; DARF: creatinine >5 mg/dL: not rec

Ibandronate	EHL 37-157 h, PRC C, Lact
Boniva Tab 2.5 mg, 150 mg, Inj 3 mg/3 mL	**Postmenopausal osteoporosis:** 2.5 mg PO qd or 150 mg qmo or 3 mg IV q3 mo; DARF GFR (mL/min) >30: 100%; <30: not rec

Pamidronate	EHL no data, Q0 0.5, PRC D, Lact ?
Aredia *Inj 30 mg/vial, 90 mg/vial* **Generics** *Inj 30 mg/vial, 90 mg/vial; 30 mg/ 10 mL, 60 mg/10 mL, 90 mg/10 mL*	**Moderate hypercalcemia** (Ca = 12-13.5 mg/ dL): 60-90 mg IV over 24 h as single dose; **severe hypercalcemia** (Ca >13.5 mg/dL): 90 mg IV single dose over 24 h, rep. prn after at least 7 d; **Paget's disease**: 30 mg IV over 4 h qd for 3 d; **osteolytic bone lesions**: 90 mg IV over 4 h q4 wk; DARF: not req in patients who receive 90 mg monthly
Risedronate	EHL 1.5 h, PRC C, Lact ?
Actonel *Tab 5 mg, 30 mg, 35 mg, 75 mg, 150 mg* **Atelvia** *Tab 35 mg*	**Paget's disease**: 30 mg PO qd for 2 mo; **postmenopausal and steroid-induced osteoporosis**: 5mg PO qd or 35 mg qwk; **osteoporosis in men**: 35 mg PO qwk; DARF: GFR (mL/min): >30: 100%, <30: not rec
Tiludronate	EHL 43-150 h, PRC C, Lact ?
Skelid *Tab 200 mg*	**Paget's disease**: 400 mg PO qd for 3 mo; DARF: GFR (mL/min): >30: 100%,<30: not rec
Zoledronate	EHL 1.5 h, Q0 0.1, PRC D, Lact -
Reclast *Inj 5 mg/100 mL* **Zometa** *Inj 4 mg/vial, 4 mg/5 mL, 4 mg/100 mL*	**Hypercalcemia of malignancy, multiple myeloma, osteolytic bone lesions**: 4 mg IV over 15 min, rep. q3-4 wk; **Paget's disease**: 5 mg over 15 min IV;

10.10.2 Calcitonin

MA/EF: calcium and phosphate uptake in bone ↑, renal calcium and phosphate excretion ↑
AE: feeling of warmth (flushing), N/V, diarrhea, rash, depression, flu-like symptoms; 2013 FDA warns about possible ↑ cancer risk
CI: hypocalcemia, hypersensitivity to salmon calcitonin products

Calcitonin-Salmon	EHL 1 h, Q0 0.9, PRC C, Lact ?
Fortical *Spray (nasal) 200 IU/spray* **Miacalcin** *Spray (nasal) 200 IU/mL, Inj 200 IU/mL*	**Postmenopausal osteoporosis**: 100 U SC/IM qd or qod; 200 U intranasal qd; **Paget's disease**: 50-100 U SC/IM qd or qod; **hypercalcemia**: 4 U/kg SC/IM q12 h, incr prn to max 8 U/kg q6-12 h

10.10.3 Calcimimetic agents

MA: increases the sensitivity of the calcium-sensing receptor to activation by extracellular calcium **EF**: lowers PTH-level and subsequently serum calcium levels
AE: N/V, diarrhea, myalgia, dizziness, hypertension, asthenia, anorexia, chest pain
CI: hypersensitivity to C.

Cinacalcet	EHL 30-40 h PRC C, Lact ?
Sensipar *Tab 30 mg, 60 mg, 90 mg*	**Sec. Hyperparathyroidism**: ini 30 mg PO qd, adjust dose q2-4wk based on PTH-level to 60-180 mg qd; **Parathyroid carcinoma**: ini 30 mg PO bid, titrate q2-4 wk up to 360 mg/day based serum calcium level; DARF: not req

10.10.4 Phosphate binding substances

MA (lanthanum): lanthanum ions bind dietary phosphate in the upper GI tract
MA (sevelamer): polymer, free of calcium and aluminum; **EF**: inhibition of enteral phosphate resorption; **AE (lanthanum c.)**: headache, hypotension, rhinitis, abdominal pain, constipation, diarrhea, nausea, vomiting, hypercalcemia, bronchitis, dialysis graft complication, dialysis graft occlusion; **AE (sevelamer)**: pain, N/V, diarrhea, constipation, flatulence, dyspepsia, dyspnea; **CI (sevelamer)**: hypophosphatemia, ileus, bowel obstruction, hypersensitivity to sevelamer products

Lanthanum carbonate	PRC C, Lact ?
Fosrenol *Tab (chew) 250 mg, 500 mg, 750 mg, 1 g*	**Hyperphosphatemia**: ini 750-1500 mg/day PO in div doses taken with meals, titrate dose q2-3 wk based on serum phosphate level, maint usually 1.5-3 g/day

Sevelamer	PRC C, Lact ?
Renagel *Tab 400 mg, 800 mg*	**Hyperphosphatemia**: 800 mg PO tid if serum-phosphate = 6-7.5 mg/dL; 1200-1600 mg PO tid if 7.5-9 mg/dL; 1600 mg PO tid if >9 mg/dL; max 4 g/dose

10.10.5 Potassium binding resins

MA: enteral application of an insoluble synthetic material with sulphonic acid as basic structure; exchange of cations for neutralization of acid according to the cation concentrations in the intestinal lumen ⇒ binding and removal of potassium; **AE:** colonic necrosis, electrolyte abnormalities, constipation, hypocalcemia, N/V; **CI:** hypersensitivity to sodium polystyrene sulfonate, hypokalemia, conditions associated with hypercalcemia, bowel obstruction

Polystyrene sulfonate	PRC C, Lact +
Kayexalate *Powder (oral, rect) 453.6 g/bot* **Kionex** *Powder (oral, rect) 454 g/bot* **SPS** *Susp (oral, rect) 15 g/60 mL* **Generics** *Susp (oral, rect) 15 g/60 mL, Powder (oral, rect) 454 g/bot*	**Hyperkalemia:** 15 g PO qd-qid; 30–50 g retention enema q6 h, retain for at least 30–60 min

10.10.6 Vasopressin antagonists

MA: antagonizes arginine-vasopressin receptors ⇒ free water excretion ↑
AE: thirst, headache, osmotic demyelination syndrome, confusion, insomnia, fever, hypertension, orthostatic hypotension, atrial fibrillation, N/V, diarrhea, dry mouth, constipation, oral candidiasis, pollakiuria, polyuria, hematuria, UTI, anemia, dehydration, hyperglycemia, hypoglycemia, hypokalemia, hypomagnesemia, hyponatremia, pneumonia, erythema, infusion site reaction;
CI: hypersensitivity to c. , hypovolemic hyponatremia, combination w/potent CYP3A4 inhibitors (ketoconazole, itraconazole, clarithromycin, ritonavir, indinavir)

Conivaptan	EHL 5-8 h PRC C, Lact ?
Vaprisol *Inj 20 mg/4 mL*	**Euvolemic Hyponatremia (SIADS, hypothyroidism, adrenal insufficiency, pulmonary disorders):** ini 20 mg over 30 min IV, then 20 mg over 24 h for 1-3 d, incr prn to max 40 mg/day, duration max 4 d

10.11 Vitamins

10.11.1 Vitamin B group

AE (thiamine/vitamin B1): IV injection site reaction; **AE** (riboflavin/vitamin B2): urine discoloration; **AE** (pyridoxine/vit. B6): neuropathy, N/V; **CI**: hypersensitivity to product ingredients; **CI** (cyanocobalamin/vitamin B12): diarrhea, urticaria, pruritus, rash

Vitamin B1 (Thiamine)	EHL , PRC A, Lact +
Generics *Tab 25 mg, 50 mg, 100 mg, 500 mg, Inj 100 mg/mL*	**RDA:** 1–1.6 mg PO qd; **Wernicke's encephalopathy:** ini 100 mg IV, then 50–100 mg IV/IM qd; **beriberi:** 10–20 mg IM tid x 2 wk, then 5–30 mg PO qd; **wet beriberi with heart failure:** 10–30 mg IV tid

Vitamin B2 (Riboflavin)	EHL 1.4h, PRC A, Lact +
Generics *Tab 10 mg*	**RDA:** 1.2–1.8 mg PO qd; **riboflavin deficiency:** 5–25 mg/day PO qd

Vitamin B6 (Pyridoxine)	EHL 15–20d, PRC A, Lact +
Generics *Tab 10 mg, 25 mg, 50 mg, 100 mg, 250 mg*	**RDA:** 1.6–2.5 mg PO qd; **pyridoxine deficiency:** 10–20 mg PO qd for 3 wk, then 2–5 mg PO qd; **PRO of isoniazid neuropathy:** 25–50 mg PO qd; **Tx of isoniazid neuropathies:** 50–200 mg PO qd

Vitamin B12 (Cyanocobalamin)	PRC A, Lact +
Rubramin PC *Inj 1 mg/mL* **Vibiseb** *Inj 1 mg/mL* **Generics** *Tab 1 mg, Inj 0.1 mg/mL, 1 mg/mL*	**RDA:** 2 mcg PO qd; **vitamin B12 deficiency:** 25–350 mcg qd PO/intranasal; **pernicious anemia:** 100 mcg/day IM/SC for 6–7 d, then 100 mcg/day IM/SC qod for 7 d, then 100 mcg/day IM/SC q3–4 d for 2–3 wk, then 100 mcg qmo IM/SC

10.11.2 Vitamin C

AE: occasional osmotic diarrhea, kidney stones, renal insufficiency; **CI:** restricted use in oxaluric urolithiasis, thalassemia and hemochromatosis, hypersensitivity to vitamin C products

Vitamin C (Ascorbic Acid)	EHL , Q0 0.3, PRC C, Lact ?
Tab 100 mg, 250 mg, 500 mg, Inj 500 mg/mL	**RDA:** 60–95 mg/day PO; **scurvy:** 300 mg/day IV/PO for 7 day, then 100 mg PO qd

10.11.3 Vitamin D

AE (calcitriol): hypercalcemia, N/V, polydipsia, polyuria; **AE** (dihydrotachysterol): hypercalcemia, renal impairment, N/V; **AE** (doxercalciferol): headache/malaise, edema, dyspnea, hypercalcemia; **CI** (calcitriol): hypercalcemia, vitamin D toxicity, hypersensitivity to calcitriol products; **CI** (dihydrotachysterol): hypercalcemia, hypersensitivity to dihydrotachysterol products; **CI** (doxercalciferol): hypercalcemia or vitamin D toxicity

Calcitriol	EHL 5-8 h, PRC C, Lact ?
Calcijex *Inj 1 mcg/mL, 2 mcg/mL,* *Sol (oral) 2 mcg/mL* **Rocaltrol** *Cap 0.5 mcg,* *Sol (oral) 1 mcg/mL* **Generics** *Cap 0.25 mcg, 0.5 mcg; Inj 1 mcg/* *mL, 2 mcg/mL*	**Hypocalcemia in dialysis patients:** ini 0.25 mcg PO qd, incr by 0.25 mcg q4-8 wk until normocalcemic, most dialysis patients respond to 0.5-1 mcg/day PO or 1-2 mcg IV tiw; **hypoparathyroidism:** 0.25 mcg PO qd; incr prn q2-4 wk up to 2 mcg/day

Dihydrotachysterol (Vitamin D)	EHL no data, PRC C, Lact ?
DHT *Tab 0.125 mg, 0.2 mg, 0.4 mg* *Sol (oral) 0.2 mg/5 mL*	**Hypoparathyroidism:** ini 0.8-2.4 mg PO qd for several days; maint 0.2-1 mg PO qd

Doxercalciferol	EHL alpha,25-(OH)2D2 32-37 h, PRC B, Lact ?
Hectorol *Cap 0.5 mcg, 1 mcg, 2.5 mcg,* *Inj 2 mcg/mL, 4 mcg/mL*	**Secondary hyperparathyroidism, dialysis patients:** 2.5-20 mcg PO tiw; 1-6 mcg IV tiw

10.11.4 Vitamin D analogs

AE: N/V; **CI:** hypersensitivity to vitamin D analogs, hypercalcemia, vitamin D toxicity

Paricalcitol	EHL 5-7 h, PRC C, Lact ?
Zemplar *Cap 1 mcg, 2 mcg, 4 mcg;* *Inj. 2 mcg/mL, 5 mcg/mL*	**Secondary hyperparathyroidism:** 0.04-0.1 mcg/kg IV tiw; iPTH <500: 1 mg PO qd or 2 mcg IV tiw; iPTH >500: 2 mcg PO qd or 4 mcg tiw; adjust dose based on iPTH-levels

10.11.5 Vitamin E

AE: bleeding DO
CI: hypersensitivity to vit. E products, IV use in low birth-weight infants, caution in coagulation DO or anticoagulation, topical use in recent chemical peel or dermabrasion

Tocopherol (Vitamin E)	EHL , PRC A, Lact +
Generics *Tab, Cap, Susp, Oint*	**RDA:** 8-10 mg PO qd; **vitamin E deficiency:** 4-5 times the RDA

10.11.6 Vitamin K

AE: when given intravenously anaphylactic reactions with apnea, dermatitis at injection site, hemolytic anemia with excessive doses; **CI:** hypersensitivity to Vitamin K, menadione (K3) administration in individuals with glucose-6-phosphate dehydrogenase deficiency

Phytonadione (Vitamin K)	EHL 26-193 h, Q0 0.95, PRC C, Lact +
Aquamephyton *Inj 1 mg/0.5 mL, 10 mg/mL* Mephyton *Tab 5 mg* Vitamin K1 *Inj 1 mg/0.5 mL, 10 mg/mL* Generics *Inj 1 mg/0.5 mL*	Hypoprothrombinemia: 2.5-25 mg PO/IM/SC; **anticoagulant-induced hypoprothrombinemia:** 2.5-10 mg PO/SC/IM; **hemorrhagic disease of the newborn:** PRO: 0.5-1 mg IM 1h after birth; Tx: 1 mg SC/IM

10.11.7 Folic acid

MA: required for nucleoprotein synthesis
AE: occasional CNS impairment, GI impairment, irritability, urticaria, pruritus
CI: megaloblastic anemia due to vit. B_{12} deficiency, hypersensitivity to folic acid products

Folic acid	EHL , PRC A, Lact +
Folicet *Tab 1 mg* Folvite *Inj 5 mg/mL* Generics *Tab 1 mg, Inj 5 mg/mL*	RDA: 0.18-0.4 mg PO qd; **megaloblastic anemia:** 1 mg PO/IM/SC/IV qd

11 Lab Values

11.1 Blood Chemistry

Test	Reference range
(A-a) O_2	5–20 mmHg
5'-Nucleotidase	2–16 U/L [0.03–0.27 µkat/L]
α_1-Antitryp. [S]	100–200 mg/dL [1–2 g/L]
ACE[S]	8–40 U/L
Acetoacetate [P]	0.2–1.0 mg/dL
Acetone [S]	<3.0 mg/dL
Acetylcholine receptor antibody	<0.04 nmol/L
ACTH, fasting [S]	<60 pg/mL [<13.2 pmol/L]
ADH	1.5–5 pg/mL [1.38–4.62 pmol/L]
AFP [S]	0.0–8.5 ng/mL
Albumin	3.5–5.3 g/dL
Aldolase [S]	0–8 U/L
Aldosterone	3–10 ng/dL (supine)
Alkaline phosphatase	40–115 U/L
Alkaline phosphatase, bone specific	14.2–42.7 U/L
ALT (SGPT)	9–60 IU/L
Aluminum [S]	<15 mcg/L
Ammonia	19–87 mcg/dL
Amylase [S]	<170 U/L [<2.84 µkat/L]
ANA antinuclear antibody	neg.: titre <1:20 pos.: titre ≥1:60
Androstenedione [S]	70–205 ng/dL
Anion Gap	8–12 mEq/L
Antibod. to dou-ble stranded DNA	<20% DNA bound
Antideoxyribonuclease B antibodies titre	<1:85
Antihistone antibodies	<1:16

Test	Reference range
Antihyluronidase titre	<128 U/mL
Antimicrosomal antibodies	0–2.0 IU/mL
Antimitochondrial antibodies	<1.0 Units
Antistreptolysin O titre	<330 IU/mL
Apolipoprotein A-I	90–160 mg/dL [0.90–1.60 g/L]
Apolipoprotein B	55–133 mg/dL [0.55–1.33 g/L]
Arsenic	2–23 mcg/L
AST (SGOT)	10–35 IU/L
Base (total) [S]	145–155 mEq/L
Betahydroxybutyrate [S]	<1.2 mmol/L
Bicarbonate [S]	24–30 mEq/L
Bile Acids, tot. [S]	0–10 μmol/L (fasting)
Bilirubin, tot. [S]	0.2–1.0 mg/dL [3.42–17 μmol/L]
Bilirubin, dir. [S]	0.1–0.3 mg/dL [1.7–5.1 μmol/L]
Bilirubin, ind. [S]	0.2–0.6 mg/dL [3.4–11 μmol/L]
Bleeding time	<10 min
Brucella antibodies	Negative or <1:80
BNP	<165 pg/mL [<165 ng/mL]
β-globulins	0.6–1.1 g/dL [9.3–15% of total]
β$_2$-microglobulin [S]	<2.3 mg/L
β-carotene [S]	10–85 mcg/dL
c AMP	5.0–25 nmol/L
CA 15-3 [S]	<31 U/mL
CA 19-9 [S]	<37 U/mL
CA 50 [S]	<17 U/mL
CA 549 [S]	<10–15.5 U/mL
CA 72-4 [S]	<3 U/mL
CA 125 [S]	0–35 U/mL
Cadmium [S]	0.1–0.4 mcg/dL

Test	Reference range
Calcitonin [P]	M: <11.5 pg/mL, F: <4.6 pg/mL
Calcium	8.4–10.3 mg/dL
Calcium, ionized	1.1–1.3 mmol/L
Calcium, 24 hour urine	<250 mg
Candida antibodies	<1:320
Carbon dioxide, tot.[S]	22–28 mEq/L [22–28 mmol/L]
Carboxyhemoglobin	0–2.3% Hb
Carboxyhemo-globin, toxic	>20% Hb
Carotene	90–200 mcg/dL [0.89–3.72 µmol/L]
Carotenoids	50–300 mcg/dL [0.9–5.6 µmol/L]
Catecholamines [P]	150–650 pg/mL
Cathepsin D	<30 pmol/mg CP
CD4/CD8 ratio	1:3.5
CD4	450–1400/mL
CD8	190–725/mL
CDT	<6 units %
CEA [S]	0–3.8 ng/mL
Smoker	0–5.5 ng/mL
Ceruloplasm. [S]	16–66 mg/dL [160–660 mg/L]
CH_{50}	19–60.0 U/mL
Chloride	98–110 mmol/L
Cholesterol	<200 mg/dL
Cholinesterase [P]	3200–6600 IU/L
Chorionic gonado-tropin (b-hCG)	<4.0 mIU/mL [<4 IU/L]
Chromium	<1.4 mcg/L
Circulating immune complexes	<0.01 g/L
Citrate [S+P]	1.7–3.0 mg/dL
Citrulline [P]	0.2–1.0 mg/dL [12–55 µmol/L]
CK [S]	M: 15–105 U/L, F: 10–80 U/L
CK- BB	0–3% of total CK

Test	Reference range
CK- MM	90–97% of total CK
CK-MB (Heart) [S]	0.3–4.9 ng/mL
Clotting time	5–15 min
Cobalt	4.0–10.0 mcg/L
Complem. C1q	9–22 mg/dL
Complem. C1r	0.025–0.10 mg/mL
Complem. C1s	0.05–0.10 g/L
Complem. C2	1.6–3.6 mg/dL
Complem. C3 [S]	88–201 mg/dL
Complem. C4 [S]	16–47 mg/dL
Complem. C5	4.8–18.5 mg/dL
Complem. C6	28–60 mcg/mL
Complem. C7	27–80 mcg/mL
Complem. C8	40–106 mcg/mL
Complem. C9	33–250 mcg/mL
Copper	70–155 mcg/dL
Cortisol, AM [P] Cortisol, PM [P]	4.3–22.4 mcg/dL [118–618 nmol/L] 3–16.6 mcg/dL [85–458 nmol/L]
C-peptide [S]	0.78–1.89 ng/mL (0.26–0.62 nmol/L)
Creatinine [S]	0.5–1.2 mg/dL
Creatine kinase [S]	**M:** 15–105 U/L, **F:** 10–80 U/L
MB fraction	0–12 U/L [0–0.20 µkat/L]
CRP [S]	<0.5 mg/dL
Cyclosporine [S]	100–400 ng/mL (83–333 nmol/L)
Cyfra 21–1	<3.3 ng/mL
Cystatin C	0.5–1.0 mg/L
Cytomegalobody antibody titer	Negative
D-dimer	<0.4 mcg/mL
δ-aminolevulinic acid [S]	15–23 mcg/dL (1.1–8.0 µmol/L)
DHEA-S [S]	50–450 mcg/dL (1.6–12.2 µmol/L)
Digoxin [P]	0.5–2.0 ng/mL (0.6–2.6 nmol/L)

Test	Reference range
Dopamine	<87 pg/mL (<475 pmol/L)
D-xylose [25 g dose]	2 h: >30 mg/dL [>2.11 mmol/L]
Elastase	60–110 ng/mL
Epinephrine	0–140 pg/mL
Erythrocyte survival rate (51Cr)	≤2 hrs
Erythropoetin	5-36 IU/L
Ethanol	<20 mg/dL
Factor I	200-400 mg/dL
Factor II	70%–120%
Factor V	70%–120%
Factor VII	70%–120%
Factor VIII	70%–150%
Factor X	70%–120%
Factor XI	70%–120%
Factor XII	70%–150%
Factor IX	70%–120%
Fatty acids	190–420 mg/dL
Ferritin	13-150 ng/mL
Fetal fibronectin	>0.050 mcg/mL
Fibrin degrad. pro.	<1 mg/L
Fibrinogen	180–350 mg/dL
Fibrinopeptide A	0.6-1.7 mg/mL
Fluoride	<0.05 mg/dL
Folate, RBC	499-1504 ng/mL
Folic acid	3-17 ng/mL
Free fatty acids	0.1-0.6 mEq/L
Fructosamine	35–50 mg/L [195–279 mmol/L]
Fructose	1–6 mg/dL
FSH	1–110 mIU/mL [1–110 IU/L]
γ-GT [S]	**M:** 11–50 U/L, **F:** 7–32 U/L

Test	Reference range
γ-enolase	<10 mcg/L
G6PD	7–12 U/g Hb [0.12–0.20 nkat/g Hb]
Galactokinase	12.1–39.7 mU/g Hb
Galactose	<20 mg/dL [<1.1 mmol/L]
Gastrin, fasting [S]	<100 pg/mL [<48.10 pmol/L]
GH, fasting [P]	M: <1 ng/mL, F: <10 ng/mL
Ghrelin	77.5–97 pg/mL
Glucose	65–100 mg/dL
Glutamate dehydrogenase	M: <4 U/L, F: <3 U/L
Glutathione [vB]	24–37 mg/dL [0.77–1.2 mmol/L]
Glycerol [P]	0.29–1.7 mg/dL [0.03–0.18 mmol/L]
Gold [S]	<10 mcg/dL [<0.51 nmol/L]
Haptoglobin 1 [S]	30–200 mg/dL
HBDH, alpha [S]	140–350 U/L
HDL cholesterol	>40 mg/dL M: <45 mg/dL, F: <55 mg/dL
Hematocrit	35%–44%
Hemoglobin A1c	4.8%–5.6%
Hemopexin	50–115 mg/dL
Heparin	Ther. range: 0.2–0.8 U/mL
Homocysteine	5–12 µmol/L
Immungl. IgA [S]	85–385 mg/dL
IgD	0–8 mg/dL
IgE	<25 mcg/dL
IgG	700–1600 mg/dL
IgM	40–230 mg/dL
IGF-1	130–450 ng/mL [18–60 nmol/L]
Insulin [S]	3–26 µIU/mL [20.84–180 pmol/L]
Iodine [S]	55–75mcg/L [433–591 nmol/L]
Iron	35–155 mcg/dL
Iron binding capacity	250–450 mcg/dL

Test	Reference range
Iron Saturation	15%–55%
Ketones tot. [S]	0.5–3.0 mg/dL
Lactic Acid [P]	5–15 mg/dL [0.6–1.7 mmol/L]
LAP [S]	**M:** 80–200 U/mL, **F:** 75–185 U/mL
LASA (lipid asso. sialic acid) [S]	<25 mg/dL
LDH [S]	100–190 U/L [1.67–3.17 µmol/L]
LDL cholesterol	<130 mg/dL (<150 mg/dL [<3.88 mmol/L])
Lead [vB]	<10 mcg/dL [<0.48 µmol/L]
Leucin [P]	<3 mg/dL [<228 µmol/L]
Leucin aminopeptidase	M: 80–200 U/mL, F: 75–180 U/mL
LH	5–150 mIU/mL
Lipase [S]	10–220 U/dL [0.4–8.34 µkat/L]
Lipoprotein (a) [S]	<30 mg/dL [1.07 µmol/L]
Lysozyme [S, P]	0.4–1.3 mg/dL [4–13 mg/L]
Macroglobulins (tot.)	70–430 mg/dL [0.7–4.3 g/L]
Magnesium	1.5–2.4 mg/dL
Malate dehydrogenase (MDH)	50–100 U/L
Manganese	<1.1 µg/L
Melatonin [S]	10–15 ng/L [45–66 pmol/L]
Mercury [S]	<5 mcg/L [<25 nmol/L]
Methionine [P]	<0.1–0.6 mg/dL [6–40 µmol/L]
Methylmalonic acid	73–376 nmol/L
Molybdenum	1.5 mcg/L
Mucin like antigen (MCA)	<17 U/L
Myoglobin	16–80 mcg/L [0.91–4.57 nmol/L]
Neopterine [S]	<2.5 ng/mL
Neutral lipids	0–150 mg/dL
Nickel	1.0–25.0 mcg/L [17–425 nmol/L]

Test	Reference range
Norepinephrine [P]	185–400 pg/mL [1093–2364 pmol/L]
N-telopeptide, urine	10–110 BCE/mmol creat
Ornithine carbamoyl transferase	0–16 U/L
Osmolality [P]	285–295 mOsm/kg
Osteocalcin	3–13 ng/mL [3–13 mcg/L]
Oxalate [S]	1.0–2.4 mcg/mL [11–27 µmol/L]
Oxytocin [P]	1.25–5 mg/mL [1–4 pmol/L]
Pancreatic elastase1	<3.5 ng/mL
Pancreatic polypeptide	<228–332 pg/mL
Pantothenic acid	1.57 to 2.66 µmol/L
Parathyroid hormone/Parathormon [P]	<2000 pg/mL
Parathyroid hormone, intact	7–53 pg/mL
Pepsinogen [S]	25–100 ng/mL
pH	7.35–7.45
Phenylalanine [S]	0.8–1.8 mg/dL
Phosphatase, alk. [S]	30–120 U/L [0.63–2.1 µkat/L]
Phosphatase, acid. [S]	0–4.3 U/L [0–71.6 nkat/L]
Phosphate[S]	3–4.5 mg/dL [0.97–1.45 mmol/L]
Phosphohexose isomerase [S]	15–67 U/L
Phospholipase A [S]	<10 U/L
Phospholipids [S]	190–320 mg/dL
Phosphorus [S]	2.7–4.7 mg/dL [0.57–1.82 mmol/L]
Porphyrins	16–60 mcg/dL
Potassium	3.5–5.5 mmol/L
Prealbumin	20–40 mg/dL
Procalcitonin	<0.5 ng/mL
Procollagen- III-peptide [S]	3.0–15.0 ng/mL
Progesterone	1–20 ng/mL
Prolactin	**M:** 0–20 ng/mL, **F:** 0–23 ng/mL

Test	Reference range
Protein, tot. [S]	6.4–8.3 g/dL
Albumin	3.1–5.4 g/dL (50–60%)
Globulins, tot	2.3–3.4 g/dL (40–50%)
α_1-Globulins	0.1–0.4 g/dL (4.2–7.2%)
α_2-Globulins	0.4–1.1 g/dL (6.8–12%)
β-Globulins	0.5–1.2 g/dL (9.3–15%)
γ-Globulins	0.7–1.7 g/dL (13–23%)
PSA [S]	<4 ng/mL
Pyruvate [P]	0.5–1.5 mg/dL [60–170 µmol/L]
Pyruvate kinase	13–17 U/g Hb
RA factor	<1:20
Renin activity [P]	0.9–3.3 ng/mL/h
Ristocetin cofactor activity	50%–150%
SCC antigen	<2.0 ng/mL
Selenium	100–340 µg/L
Serotonin	50–200 ng/L [0.28–1.14 µmol/L]
Sodium	135–145 mmol/L
Soluble transferrin receptor	8.7–28 nmol/L
Somatomedin C	130–450 ng/mL [16–60 nmol/L]
Somatostatin [P]	<25 pg/mL [<15 pmol/L]
Sorbite dehydro-genase [S]	<0.4 U/L
Sulfate inorg.	0.2–1.3 mval/L
T_4, tot. [S]	4.5–12 mcg/dL [58–155 nmol/L]
free T_4 [S]	0.8–2.4 ng/dL [10–31 pmol/L]
T_3, tot. [S]	110–230 ng/dL [1.2–1.5 nmol/L]
T_3 uptake [S]	24–34%
T3 reverse	13–50 ng/dL
T helper (CD4)	28%–57%
T- suppr. (CD8)	10%–39%
Testosterone (male)	348–1197 ng/dL
Thallium	<10 ng/mL [<48 nmol/L]
Thiocyanate [S]	Non-smoker: 1–4 mcg/mL

Test	Reference range
Thromb. clot. time	15–18 sec
Thyroglobulin [S]	3–42 ng/mL
Thyroidal iodine (^{123}I) uptake	5%–30% of administered dose at 24 h
Thyrotropin releasing horm [P]	5–60 pg/mL
Thyroxine binding globulin	13.0–30.0 mcg/mL [222–512 nmol/L]
tPA [P]	<0.04 IU/mL [<40 IU/L]
TPA	<80 U/L
Transferrin [S]	215–380 mg/dL [2.64–4.5 µmol/L]
Transferr. saturat.	30–40%
Triglycerides	<150 mg/dL
Troponin I	<0.05 ng/L
Normal	<0.7 ng/mL
Indeterminant	0.7–1.5 ng/mL
Abnormal	>1.5 ng/mL
Troponin T	<0.1 ng/mL
Tryptophan	0.51–1.49 mg/dL [24–72 µmol/L]
Trypsin	5.0–85.0 mcg/L
TSH [S]	0.3–4.2 mIU/L
Urea [S]	17–42 mg/dL [6.0–15 mmol/L]
Urea nitrogen	7–23 ng/dL
Uric acid	2.4–8.2 mg/dL
Vasoactive intestinal polypeptide [P]	<50 pg/mL
Vitamin A (Retinol), Serum or Plasma	0.1–0.3 mg/L
Vitamin A	19–83 mcg/dL
Vitamin B1 (Thiamine), Plasma	8–30 nmol/L
Vitamin B2 (Riboflavin)	5–50 nmol/L
Vitamin B6 (Pyridoxal 5-Phosphate)	20–125 nmol/l
Vitamin B12	193–982 pg/mL
Vitamin C	0.4–2 mg/dL
Vitamin D, 25 hydroxy	32–100 ng/mL
Vitamin E	3.0–15.8 mg/L

Test	Reference range
Vitamin K	0.15–3.5 ng/mL
Zinc	70–150 mcg/dL

11.2 Hematology

Test	Reference range
Hemoglobin	**M:** 13.5–17.5, **F:** 12–16 (g/dL)
Methemoglobin	<2% of total
Hematocrit	**M:** 42–52, **F:** 37–47 (%)
Erythrocyt. count	M: 4.5–5.7, F: 3.9–5.0 (x10^6/µL)
MCV	80–100 µ
MCH	26–34 pg/cell
MCHC	31–37 g/dL
Reticulocytes	Adults/Children: 0.5%–2%
	Infants: 0.5%–3.1%
Leukocytes, tot.	4.5–11 (x10^3/µL; 100%)
Neutrophils	1.8–7.7 (x10^3/µL; 59%)
Bands	<8%
Segmented	1.8–7.0 (x10^3/µL; 56%)
Eosinophils	0–0.45 (x10^3/µL; 2.7%)
Basophils	0–0.2 (x10^3/µL; 0.5%)
Lymphocytes	1.0–4.8 (x10^3/µL; 34%)
B-cell	6%–19%
T-cell	55%–83%
T-Helper (CD4)	28%–57%
T-Suppr. (CD8)	10%–39%
CD4/CD8-rat.	1.0–3.6
Monocytes	0.2–0.9 (x10^3/µL); (**4%**)
Thrombocyt. cou.	150–400 (x10^3/µL)
AT III	Functional: 80%–120% Immunologic: 17–30 mg/dL

Test	Reference range
Bleeding Time Duke: Ivy: Simplate:	 1–4 min (<4 min) 2–7 min (5 mm wound <9min) 2.75–8.00 min
ESR Wintrobe	**M:** 0–9 mm/h, **F:** 0–20 mm/h, **CH:** 0–13 mm/h
Fibrinogen	150–400 mg/dL
Fibrin.degrad.pro.	<1:25
Prothrombin time	11–14 s
Part.Thro.pla.time	27–40 s
Thrombin time	15–18 s
Viscosity [P, S]	P:1.7–2.1 (H_2O) S:1.4–1.8 (H_2O)

11.3 Urine and Urinalysis

Test	Reference range
Acetone	0.3–2.0 mg/dL
Albumin	50–80 mg/24h (at rest)
Aldosterone	2–26 mcg/day (6–72 nmol/day)
Ammonia	30–50 mEq/day (30–50 mmoL/d)
Amylase	0–18 U/h
Beta 2 microglobulin	<120 mcg/24 hours (<10 mmol/day)
Bilirubin	negative
Blood, occult	negative
Cadmium	0.5–4.7 mcg/L
Calcium	100–300 mg/day
Calculated albumin excretion rate	at rest: 2–80 mg/24hrs ambulatory: <150 mg/24 hrs in child <10 yrs: <100mg/24 hrs
cAMP	112–188 mg/L
Chloride	150–250 mEq/day
Copper	15–60 mcg/day
Coproporphyrin	100–300 mcg/day [150–460 nmol/day]

Test	Reference range
Cortisol, free	10–100 mcg/day [27–276 nmol/day]
Creatinine	M: 0.7–1.2 g/day, F: 0.6–1.1 mg/day
Cystine/Cysteine	10–100 mg/day [0.08–0.83 mmol/day]
δ-Aminolevulinic acid	1–7 mg/24h [0.1–0.6 mg/dL]
Dopamine	60–400 mcg/day
Epinephrine	<0–15 mcg/day [0–82 nmol/day]
Erythrocytes	<3 cells/hpf
Estriol	M: 0.3–2.4 mg/24hrs, F: 0–54 mg/24hrs
Estrogens	M: 4–23 g/g creatinine, F: 7–135 g/g creatinine
Fat	negative
Fructose	30–65 mg/h
FSH	M: >2–18 IU/24hrs, F: 2–100 IU/24hrs
GFR	125 mL/min
Glucose	<0.5 g/d [<2.78 mmol/day]
hCG	Negative or <3.0 mIU/mL
Homocysteine	0–9 μmol/g of creatinine
Homovanillic acid (HVA)	<8 mg/24hrs (10–35 mol/24hrs)
5-HIAA	2–6 mg/day [10.4–31.2 μmol/day]
Hydroxyproli. tot	15–45 mg/day
Ketones total	negative
17-keto steroids	M: 7–25 mg/day [24–88 μmol/day], F: 4–15 mg/day [14–52 μmol/day]
17-OCHS	M:4.5–10 mg/day, F: 2.5–10 mg/day
Legionella antigen	Negative
Leukocyte esterase	Negative
Leukocytes	≤4 cells/hpf
Luteinizing hormone	M: 5–25 IU/24 h F: 2–100 IU/24 h
Magnesium	5–16 mEq/day [0.5–12 mmol/day]
Melanin	Negative

Test	Reference range
MSH	Negative
Mercury	0–10 mcg/L
Metanephrine	24–96 mcg/day
Muramidase	<3 mcg/mL (0–2.9 mg/L)
Nitrite	Negative
Norepinephrine	15–80 mcg/day [88.5–472 nmol/day]
Osmolality 12h fluid rest	50–1400 mOsmol/kg >850 mOsmol/kg/day
Oxalate	**M:** 7–44 mg/day [80–502 μmol/day], **F:** 4–31 mg/day [46–353 μmol/day]
Pentoses	2.0–5.0 mg/kg/24h
pH	4.8–7.5
Phosphorus	0.4–1.3 g/day [13–42 mmol/day]
Porphobilinogen	0–2.0 mg/day [0–8.8 μmol/day]
Porphyrins Coproporphyrin	**M:** <97 mcg/day, **F:** <61 mcg/day
Uroporphyrin	**M:** <47 mcg/day, **F:** <23 mcg/day
Potassium	25–125 mEq/day
Protein, total	<150 mg/dL [<856 mg/day at rest]
Sodium	80–200 mEq/L/day
Spec. Gravit. rand.	1.005–1.030
Thallium	<2 mcg/L
Trypsinogen–2	<50 ng/mL
U,12h fluid restric.	>1.025
U, 24	1.015–1.025
Urea-Nitrogen	6–17 g/24 h [0.21–0.60 mol/day]
Uric acid	250–750 mg/day [1.5–4.5 mmol/day]
Urinary gonado-trophin peptide	<0.2 ng/mL
Urobilinogen	1–3.5 mg24 h
VMA	2.0–7.0 mg/day
Volume	600–2500 mL/day

11.4 Stool

Test	Reference range
Fat	<6 g/day (2.5–5.5 g/24 h) (<30.4% of dry weight)
Trypsin Activity	positive (2+ to 4+)
Pancreatic elastase 1	200–500 mcg/g
Wet Weight	<197.5 g/day (74–155 g/day)
Dry Weight	<66.4 g/day (18–50 g/day)

12 Dietary Reference Intakes (DRIs)

(see reference [103])

12.1 Estimated Average Requirements

Life stage group	Calcium (mg/d)	CHO (g/d)	Protein (g/kg/d)	Vitamin A (mcg/d)[a]	Vitamin C (mg/d)	Vitamin D (mcg/d)	Vitamin E (mg/d)[b]	Thiamin (mg/d)	Riboflavin (mg/d)	Niacin (mg/d)[e]	Vitamin B$_6$ (mg/d)
Infants											
0–6 mo	–	–	–	–	–	–	–	–	–	–	–
6–12 mo	–	–	1.0	–	–	–	–	–	–	–	–
Children											
1–3 y	500	100	0.87	210	13	10	5	0.4	0.4	5	0.4
4–8 y	800	100	0.76	275	22	10	6	0.5	0.5	6	0.5
Male											
9–13 y	1,100	100	0.76	445	39	10	9	0.7	0.8	9	0.8
14–18 y	1,100	100	0.73	630	63	10	12	1.0	1.1	12	1.1
19–30 y	800	100	0.66	625	75	10	12	1.0	1.1	12	1.1
31–50 y	800	100	0.66	625	75	10	12	1.0	1.1	12	1.1
51–70 y	800	100	0.66	625	75	10	12	1.0	1.1	12	1.4
>70 y	1,000	100	0.66	625	75	10	12	1.0	1.1	12	1.4
Female											
9–13 y	1,100	100	0.76	420	39	10	9	0.7	0.8	9	0.8
14–18 y	1,100	100	0.71	485	56	10	12	0.9	0.9	11	1.0
19–30 y	800	100	0.66	500	60	10	12	0.9	0.9	11	1.1
31–50 y	800	100	0.66	500	60	10	12	0.9	0.9	11	1.1
51–70 y	1,000	100	0.66	500	60	10	12	0.9	0.9	11	1.3
>70 y	1,000	100	0.66	500	60	10	12	0.9	0.9	11	1.3
Pregnancy											
14–18 y	1,000	135	0.88	530	66	10	12	1.2	1.2	14	1.6
19–30 y	800	135	0.88	550	70	10	12	1.2	1.2	14	1.6
31–50 y	800	135	0.88	550	70	10	12	1.2	1.2	14	1.6
Lactation											
14–18 y	1,000	160	1.05	885	96	10	16	1.2	1.3	13	1.7
19–30 y	800	160	1.05	900	100	10	16	1.2	1.3	13	1.7
31–50 y	800	160	1.05	900	100	10	16	1.2	1.3	13	1.7

Estimated average requirements (cont.)										
Life stage group	Folate (mcg/d)[d]	Vitamin B_{12} (mcg/d)	Copper (mcg/d)	Iodine (mcg/d)	Iron (mg/d)	Magnesium (mg/d)	Molybdenum (mcg/d)	Phosphorus (mg/d)	Selenium (mcg/d)	Zinc (mg/d)
Infants										
0–6 mo	–	–	–	–	–	–	–	–	–	–
6–12 mo	–	–	–	–	6.9	–	–	–	–	2.5
Children										
1–3 y	120	0.7	260	65	3.0	65	13	380	17	2.5
4–8 y	160	1.0	340	65	4.1	110	17	405	23	4.0
Male										
9–13 y	250	1.5	540	73	5.9	200	26	1,055	35	7.0
14–18 y	330	2.0	685	95	7.7	340	33	1,055	45	8.5
19–30 y	320	2.0	700	95	6	330	34	580	45	9.4
31–50 y	320	2.0	700	95	6	350	34	580	45	9.4
51–70 y	320	2.0	700	95	6	350	34	580	45	9.4
>70 y	320	2.0	700	95	6	350	34	580	45	9.4
Female										
9–13 y	250	1.5	540	73	5.7	200	26	1,055	35	7.0
14–18 y	330	2.0	685	95	7.9	300	33	1,055	45	7.3
19–30 y	320	2.0	700	95	8.1	255	34	580	45	6.8
31–50 y	320	2.0	700	95	8.1	265	34	580	45	6.8
51–70 y	320	2.0	700	95	5	265	34	580	45	6.8
>70 y	320	2.0	700	95	5	265	34	580	45	6.8
Pregnancy										
14–18 y	520	2.2	785	160	23	335	40	1,055	49	10.5
19–30 y	520	2.2	800	160	22	290	40	580	49	9.5
31–50 y	520	2.2	800	160	22	300	40	580	49	9.5
Lactation										
14–18 y	450	2.4	985	209	7	300	35	1,055	59	10.9
19–30 y	450	2.4	1,000	209	6.5	255	36	580	59	10.4
31–50 y	450	2.4	1,000	209	6.5	265	36	580	59	10.4

12.2 RDA and Adequate Intakes

12.2.1 Vitamins

Life stage group	Vitamin A (mcg/d)[a]	Vitamin C (mg/d)	Vitamin D (mcg/d)[b,c]	Vitamin E (mg/d)[d]	Vitamin K (mcg/d)	Thiamin (mg/d)	Riboflavin (mg/d)
Infants							
0–6 mo	400*	40*	10	4*	2.0*	0.2*	0.3*
6–12 mo	500*	50*	10	5*	2.5*	0.3*	0.4*
Children							
1–3 y	300	15	15	6	30*	0.5	0.5
4–8 y	400	25	15	7	55*	0.6	0.6
Male							
9–13 y	600	45	15	11	60*	0.9	0.9
14–18 y	900	75	15	15	75*	1.2	1.3
19–30 y	900	90	15	15	120*	1.2	1.3
31–50 y	900	90	15	15	120*	1.2	1.3
51–70 y	900	90	15	15	120*	1.2	1.3
>70 y	900	90	20	15	120*	1.2	1.3
Female							
9–13 y	600	45	15	11	60*	0.9	0.9
14–18 y	700	65	15	15	75*	1.0	1.0
19–30 y	700	75	15	15	90*	1.1	1.1
31–50 y	700	75	15	15	90*	1.1	1.1
51–70 y	700	75	15	15	90*	1.1	1.1
>70 y	700	75	20	15	90*	1.1	1.1
Pregnancy							
14–18 y	750	80	15	15	75*	1.4	1.4
19–30 y	770	85	15	15	90*	1.4	1.4
31–50 y	770	85	15	15	90*	1.4	1.4
Lactation							
14–18 y	1200	115	15	19	75*	1.4	1.6
19–30 y	1,300	120	15	19	90*	1.4	1.6
31–50 y	1,300	120	15	19	90*	1.4	1.6

| Vitamins (cont.) | | | | | | | |
Life stage group	Niacin (mg/d)[e]	Vitamin B$_6$ (mg/d)	Folate (mcg/d)[f]	Vitamin B$_{12}$ (mcg/d)	Pantothenic acid (mg/d)	Biotin (mcg/d)	Choline (mg/d)[g]
Infants							
0–6 mo	2*	0.1*	65*	0.4*	1.7*	5*	125*
6–12 mo	4*	0.3*	80*	0.5*	1.8*	6*	150*
Children							
1–3 y	6	0.5	150	0.9	2*	8*	200*
4–8 y	8	0.6	200	1.2	3*	12*	250*
Male							
9–13 y	12	1.0	300	1.8	4*	20*	375*
14–18 y	16	1.3	400	2.4	5*	25*	550*
19–30 y	16	1.3	400	2.4	5*	30*	550*
31–50 y	16	1.3	400	2.4	5*	30*	550*
51–70 y	16	1.7	400	2.4h	5*	30*	550*
>70 y	16	1.7	400	2.4h	5*	30*	550*
Female							
9–13 y	12	1.0	300	1.8	4*	20*	375*
14–18 y	14	1.2	400[i]	2.4	5*	25*	400*
19–30 y	14	1.3	400[i]	2.4	5*	30*	425*
31–50 y	14	1.3	400[i]	2.4	5*	30*	425*
51–70 y	14	1.5	400	2.4[h]	5*	30*	425*
>70 y	14	1.5	400	2.4[h]	5*	30*	425*
Pregnancy							
14–18 y	18	1.9	600[i]	2.6	6*	30*	450*
19–30 y	18	1.9	600[i]	2.6	6*	30*	450*
31–50 y	18	1.9	600[i]	2.6	6*	30*	450*
Lactation							
14–18 y	17	2.0	500	2.8	7*	35*	550*
19–30 y	17	2.0	500	2.8	7*	35*	550*
31–50 y	17	2.0	500	2.8	7*	35*	550*

12.2.2 Elements Life stage group	Calcium (mg/d)	Chromium (mcg/d)	Copper (mcg/d)	Fluoride (mg/d)	Iodine (mcg/d)	Iron (mg/d)	Magnesium (mg/d)	Manganese (mg/d)
Infants								
0-6 mo	200*	0.2*	200*	0.01*	110*	0.27*	30*	0.003*
6-12 mo	260*	5.5*	220*	0.5*	130*	11	75*	0.6*
Children								
1-3 y	700	11*	340*	0.7*	90	7	80	1.2*
4-8 y	1,000	15*	440*	1*	90	10	130	1.5*
Male								
9-13 y	1,300	25*	700	2*	120	8	240	1.9*
14-18 y	1,300	35*	890	3*	150	11	410	2.2*
19-30 y	1,000	35*	900	4*	150	8	400	2.3*
31-50 y	1,000	35*	900	4*	150	8	420	2.3*
51-70 y	1,000	30*	900	4*	150	8	420	2.3*
>70 y	1,200	30*	900	4*	150	8	420	2.3*
Female								
9-13 y	1,300	21*	700	2*	120	8	240	1.6*
14-18 y	1,300	24*	890	3*	150	15	360	1.6*
19-30 y	1,000	25*	900	3*	150	18	310	1.8*
31-50 y	1,000	25*	900	3*	150	18	320	1.8*
51-70 y	1,200	20*	900	3*	150	8	320	1.8*
>70 y	1,200	20*	900	3*	150	8	320	1.8*
Pregnancy								
14-18 y	1,300	29*	1,000	3*	220	27	400	2.0*
19-30 y	1,000	30*	1,000	3*	220	27	350	2.0*
31-50 y	1,000	30*	1,000	3*	220	27	360	2.0*
Lactation								
14-18 y	1,300	44*	1,300	3*	290	10	360	2.6*
19-30 y	1,000	45*	1,300	3*	290	9	310	2.6*
31-50 y	1,000	45*	1,300	3*	290	9	320	2.6*

Elements (cont.)							
Life stage group	Molybdenum (mcg/d)	Phosphorus (mg/d)	Selenium (mcg/d)	Zinc (mg/d)	Potassium (g/d)	Sodium (g/d)	Chloride (g/d)
Infants							
0-6 mo	2*	100*	15*	2*	0.4*	0.12*	0.18*
6-12 mo	3*	275*	20*	3	0.7*	0.37*	0.57*
Children							
1-3 y	17	460	20	3	3.0*	1.0*	1.5*
4-8 y	22	500	30	5	3.8*	1.2*	1.9*
Male							
9-13 y	34	1,250	40	8	4.5*	1.5*	2.3*
14-18 y	43	1,250	55	11	4.7*	1.5*	2.3*
19-30 y	45	700	55	11	4.7	1.5*	2.3*
31-50 y	45	700	55	11	4.7	1.5*	2.3*
51-70 y	45	700	55	11	4.7	1.3*	2.0*
>70 y	45	700	55	11	4.7	1.2*	1.8*
Female							
9-13 y	34	1,250	40	8	4.5*	1.5*	2.3*
14-18 y	43	1,250	55	9	4.7*	1.5*	2.3*
19-30 y	45	700	55	8	4.7	1.5*	2.3*
31-50 y	45	700	55	8	4.7	1.5*	2.3*
51-70 y	45	700	55	8	4.7	1.3*	2.0*
>70 y	45	700	55	8	4.7	1.2*	1.8*
Pregnancy							
14-18 y	50	1,250	60	12	4.7	1.5*	2.3*
19-30 y	50	700	60	11	4.7	1.5*	2.3*
31-50 y	50	700	60	11	4.7	1.5*	2.3*
Lactation							
14-18 y	50	1,250	70	13	5.1*	1.5*	2.3*
19-30 y	50	700	70	12	5.1*	1.5*	2.3*
31-50 y	50	700	70	12	5.1*	1.5*	2.3*

→ Food and Nutrition Board, Institute of Medicine, National Academies
NOTE: This table (taken from the DRI reports, see www.nap.edu) presents Recommended Dietary Allowances (RDAs) in **bold type** and Adequate Intakes (AIs) in ordinary type followed by an asterisk (*). An RDA is the average daily dietary intake level; sufficient to meet the nutrient requirements of nearly all (97–98 percent) healthy individuals in a group. It is calculated from an Estimated Average Requirement (EAR). If sufficient scientific evidence is not available to establish an EAR, and thus calculate an RDA, an AI is usually developed. For healthy breastfed infants, an AI is the mean intake. The AI for other life stage and gender groups is believed to cover the needs of all healthy individuals in the groups, but lack of data or uncertainty in the data prevent being able to specify with confidence the percentage of individuals covered by this intake.

a As retinol activity equivalents (RAEs). 1 RAE = 1 mg retinol, 12 mg β-carotene, 24 mg α-carotene, or 24 mg β-cryptoxanthin. The RAE for dietary provitamin A carotenoids is two-fold greater than retinol equivalents (RE), whereas the RAE for preformed vitamin A is the same as RE.

b As cholecalciferol. 1 mcg cholecalciferol = 40 IU vitamin D

c Under the assumption of minimal sunlight

d As α-tocopherol. α-Tocopherol includes RRR-α-tocopherol, the only form of α-tocopherol that occurs naturally in foods, and the 2R-stereoisomeric forms of α-tocopherol (RRR-, RSR-, RRS-, and RSS-α-tocopherol) that occur in fortified foods and supplements. It does not include the 2S-stereoisomeric forms of α-tocopherol (SRR-, SSR-, SRS-, and SSS-α-tocopherol), also found in fortified foods and supplements.

e As niacin equivalents (NE). 1 mg of niacin = 60 mg of tryptophan; 0–6 months = preformed niacin (not NE)

f As dietary folate equivalents (DFE). 1 DFE = 1 mcg food folate = 0.6 mcg of folic acid from fortified food or as a supplement consumed with food = 0.5 mcg of a supplement taken on an empty stomach

g Although AIs have been set for choline, there are few data to assess whether a dietary supply of choline is needed at all stages of the life cycle, and it may be that the choline requirement can be met by endogenous synthesis at some of these stages

h Because 10 to 30 percent of older people may malabsorb food-bound B12, it is advisable for those older than 50 years to meet their RDA mainly by consuming foods fortified with B12 or a supplement containing B12

i In view of evidence linking folate intake with neural tube defects in the fetus, it is recommended that all women capable of becoming pregnant consume 400 mcg from supplements or fortified foods in addition to intake of food folate from a varied diet

j It is assumed that women will continue consuming 400 mcg from supplements or fortified food until their pregnancy is confirmed and they enter prenatal care, which ordinarily occurs after the end of the periconceptional period—the critical time for formation of the neural tube

12.2.3 Total water and macronutrients

Life stage group	Total Water[a] (L/d)	Carbohydrate (g/d)	Total Fiber (g/d)	Fat (g/d)	Linoleic Acid (g/d)	α-Linolenic Acid (g/d)	Protein[b] (g/d)
Infants							
0–6 mo	0.7*	60*	ND	31*	4.4*	0.5*	9.1*
6–12 mo	0.8*	95*	ND	30*	4.6*	0.5*	11.0*
Children							
1–3 y	1.3*	130	19*	ND[c]	7*	0.7*	13
4–8 y	1.7*	130	25*	ND	10*	0.9*	19
Male							
9–13 y	2.4*	130	31*	ND	12*	1.2*	34
14–18 y	3.3*	130	38*	ND	16*	1.6*	52
19–30 y	3.7*	130	38*	ND	17*	1.6*	56
31–50 y	3.7*	130	38*	ND	17*	1.6*	56
51–70 y	3.7*	130	30*	ND	14*	1.6*	56
>70 y	3.7*	130	30*	ND	14*	1.6*	56
Female							
9–13 y	2.1*	130	26*	ND	10*	1.0*	34
14–18 y	2.3*	130	26*	ND	11*	1.1*	46
19–30 y	2.7*	130	25*	ND	12*	1.1*	46
31–50 y	2.7*	130	25*	ND	12*	1.1*	46
51–70 y	2.7*	130	21*	ND	11*	1.1*	46
>70 y	2.7*	130	21*	ND	11*	1.1*	46
Pregnancy							
14–18 y	3.0*	175	28*	ND	13*	1.4*	71
19–30 y	3.0*	175	28*	ND	13*	1.4*	71
31–50 y	3.0*	175	28*	ND	13*	1.4*	71
Lactation							
14–18 y	3.8*	210	29*	ND	13*	13*	71
19–30 y	3.8*	210	29*	ND	13*	13*	71
31–50 y	3.8*	210	29*	ND	13*	13*	71

12.3 Macronutrients

12.3.1 Carbohydrate—total digestible

Function	Life stage group	RDA/AI* g/d	AMDRᵃ	Selected food sources	Adverse effects of excessive consumption
RDA based on its role as the primary energy source for the brain; AMDR based on its role as a source of kilocalories to maintain body weight	**Infants**			Starch and sugar are the major types of carbohydrates. Grains and vegetables (corn, pasta, rice, potatoes, breads) are sources of starch. Natural sugars are found in fruits and juices. Sources of added sugars are soft drinks, candy, fruit drinks, and desserts.	While no defined intake level at which potential adverse effects of total digestible carbohydrate was identified, the upper end of the adequate macronutrient distribution range (AMDR) was based on decreasing risk of chronic disease and providing adequate intake of other nutrients. It is suggested that the maximal intake of added sugars be limited to providing no more than 25 percent of energy.
	0–6 mo	60*	NDᵇ		
	7–12 mo	95*	ND		
	Children				
	1–3 y	**130**	45–65		
	4–8 y	**130**	45–65		
	Male				
	9–13 y	**130**	45–65		
	14–18 y	**130**	45–65		
	19–30 y	**130**	45–65		
	31–50 y	**130**	45–65		
	50–70 y	**130**	45–65		
	>70 y	**130**	45–65		
	Female				
	9–13 y	**130**	45–65		
	14–18 y	**130**	45–65		
	19–30 y	**130**	45–65		
	31–50 y	**130**	45–65		
	50–70 y	**130**	45–65		
	>70 y	**130**	45–65		
	Pregnancy				
	≤18 y	**175**	45–65		
	19–30 y	**175**	45–65		
	31–50 y	**175**	45–65		
	Lactation				
	≤18 y	**210**	45–65		
	19–30 y	**210**	45–65		
	31–50 y	**210**	45–65		

12.3.2 Total fiber

Function	Life stage group	RDA/AI* g/d	AMDR[a]	Selected food sources	Adverse effects of excessive consumption
Improves laxation, reduces risk of coronary heart disease, assists in maintaining normal blood glucose levels.	**Infants**			Includes dietary fiber naturally present in grains (such as found in oats, wheat, or unmilled rice) and functional fiber synthesized or isolated from plants or animals and shown to be of benefit to health	Dietary fiber can have variable compositions and therefore it is difficult to link a specific source of fiber with a particular adverse effect, especially when phytate is also present in the natural fiber source. It is concluded that as part of an overall healthy diet, a high intake of dietary fiber will not produce deleterious effects in healthy individuals. While occasional adverse gastrointestinal symptoms are observed when consuming some isolated or synthetic fibers, serious chronic adverse effects have not been observed. Due to the bulky nature of fibers, excess consumption is likely to be self-' limiting. Therefore, a UL was not set for individual functional fibers.
	0-6 mo	ND	–		
	7-12 mo	ND	–		
	Children				
	1-3 y	19*	–		
	4-8 y	25*	–		
	Male				
	9-13 y	31*	–		
	14-18 y	38*	–		
	19-30 y	38*	–		
	31-50 y	38*	–		
	50-70 y	30*	–		
	>70 y	30*	–		
	Female				
	9-13 y	26*	–		
	14-18 y	26*	–		
	19-30 y	25*	–		
	31-50 y	25*	–		
	50-70 y	21*	–		
	>70 y	21*	–		
	Pregnancy				
	≤18 y	28*	–		
	19-30 y	28*	–		
	31-50 y	28*	–		
	Lactation				
	≤18 y	29*	–		
	19-30 y	29*	–		
	31-50 y	29*	–		

12.3.3 Total fat

Function	Life stage group	RDA/AI* g/d	AMDR[a]	Selected food sources	Adverse effects of excessive consumption
Energy source and when found in foods, is a source of n-6 and n-3 polyunsaturated fatty acids. Its presence in the diet increases absorption of fat soluble vitamins and precursors such as vitamin A and pro-vitamin A carotenoids.	**Infants**			Butter, margarine, vegetable oils, whole milk, visible fat on meat and poultry products, invisible fat in fish, shellfish, some plant products such as seeds and nuts, and bakery products.	While no defined intake level at which potential adverse effects of total fat was identified, the upper end of AMDR is based on decreasing risk of chronic disease and providing adequate intake of other nutrients. The lower end of the AMDR is based on concerns related to the increase in plasma triacylglycerol concentrations and decreased HDL choelesterol concentrations seen with very low fat (and thus high carbohydrate) diets
	0-6 mo	31*	–		
	7-12 mo	30*	–		
	Children				
	1-3 y	–	30-40		
	4-8 y	–	25-35		
	Male				
	9-13 y	–	25-35		
	14-18 y	–	25-35		
	19-30 y	–	20-35		
	31-50 y	–	20-35		
	50-70 y	–	20-35		
	>70 y	–	20-35		
	Female				
	9-13 y	–	25-35		
	14-18 y	–	25-35		
	19-30 y	–	20-35		
	31-50 y	–	20-35		
	50-70 y	–	20-35		
	>70 y	–	20-35		
	Pregnancy				
	≤18 y	–	20-35		
	19-30 y	–	20-35		
	31-50 y	–	20-35		
	Lactation				
	≤18 y	–	20-35		
	19-30 y	–	20-35		
	31-50 y	–	20-35		

12.3.4 n-6 Polyunsaturated fatty acids (linoleic acid)

Function	Life stage group	RDA/AI* g/d	AMDR[a]	Selected food sources	Adverse effects of excessive consumption
Essential component of structural membrane lipids, involved with cell signaling, and precursor of eicosanoids. Required for normal skin function.	**Infants**			Nuts, seeds, and vegetable oils such as soybean, safflower, and corn oil	While no defined intake level at which potential adverse effects of n-6 polyunsaturated fatty acids was identified, the upper end of the AMDR is based the lack of evidence that demonstrates long-term safety and human in vitro studies which show increased free radical formation and lipid peroxidation with higher amounts of n-6 fatty acids. Lipid peroxidation is thought to be a component of in the development of atherosclerotic plaques.
	0-6 mo	4.4*	ND[b]		
	7-12 mo	4.6*	ND		
	Children				
	1-3 y	7*	5-10		
	4-8 y	10*	5-10		
	Male				
	9-13 y	12*	5-10		
	14-18 y	16*	5-10		
	19-30 y	17*	5-10		
	31-50 y	17*	5-10		
	50-70 y	14*	5-10		
	>70 y	14*	5-10		
	Female				
	9-13 y	10*	5-10		
	14-18 y	11*	5-10		
	19-30 y	12*	5-10		
	31-50 y	12*	5-10		
	50-70 y	11*	5-10		
	>70 y	11*	5-10		
	Pregnancy				
	≤18 y	13*	5-10		
	19-30 y	13*	5-10		
	31-50 y	13*	5-10		
	Lactation				
	≤18 y	13*	5-10		
	19-30 y	13*	5-10		
	31-50 y	13*	5-10		

12.3.5 n-3 Polyunsaturated fatty acids (α-linolenic acid)

Function	Life stage group	RDA/AI* g/d	AMDR[a]	Selected food sources	Adverse effects of excessive consumption
Involved with neurological development and growth. Precursor of eicosanoids.	**Infants**			Vegetable oils such as soybean, canola, and flax seed oil, fish oils, fatty fish, with smaller amounts in meats and eggs	While no defined intake level at which potential adverse effects of n-3 polyunsaturated fatty acids was identified, the upper end of AMDR is based on maintaining the appropriate balance with n-6 fatty acids and on the lack of evidence that demonstrates long-term safety, along with human in vitro studies which show increased free-radical formation and lipid peroxidation with higher amounts of polyunsaturated fatty acids. Lipid peroxidation is thought to be a component of in the development of atherosclerotic plaques.
	0–6 mo	0.5*	ND[b]		
	7–12 mo	0.5*	ND		
	Children				
	1–3 y	0.7*	0.6–1.2		
	4–8 y	0.9*	0.6–1.2		
	Male				
	9–13 y	1.2*	0.6–1.2		
	14–18 y	1.6*	0.6–1.2		
	19–30 y	1.6*	0.6–1.2		
	31–50 y	1.6*	0.6–1.2		
	50–70 y	1.6*	0.6–1.2		
	>70 y	1.6*	0.6–1.2		
	Female				
	9–13 y	1.0*	0.6–1.2		
	14–18 y	1.1*	0.6–1.2		
	19–30 y	1.1*	0.6–1.2		
	31–50 y	1.1*	0.6–1.2		
	50–70 y	1.1*	0.6–1.2		
	>70 y	1.1*	0.6–1.2		
	Pregnancy				
	≤18 y	1.4*	0.6–1.2		
	19–30 y	1.4*	0.6–1.2		
	31–50 y	1.4*	0.6–1.2		
	Lactation				
	≤18 y	1.3*	0.6–1.2		
	19–30 y	1.3*	0.6–1.2		
	31–50 y	1.3*	0.6–1.2		

12.3.6 Saturated and trans fatty acids, and cholesterol

Function	Life stage group	RDA/AI* g/d	AMDRª	Selected food sources	Adverse effects of excessive consumption
No required role for these nutrients other than as energy sources was identified; the body can synthesize its needs for saturated fatty acids and cholesterol from other sources.	**Infants**			Saturated fatty acids are present in animal fats (meat fats and butter fat), and coconut and palm kernel oils. Sources of cholesterol include liver, eggs, and foods that contain eggs such as cheesecake and custard pies. Sources of trans fatty acids include stick margarines and foods containing hydrogenated or partiallyhydrogenated vegetable shortenings.	There is an incremental increase in plasma total and low-density lipoprotein cholesterol concentrations with increased intake of saturated or trans fatty acids or with cholesterol at even very low levels in the diet. Therefore, the intakes of each should be minimized while consuming a nutritionally adequate diet.
	0-6 mo	ND	–		
	7-12 mo	ND	–		
	Children				
	1-3 y	–	–		
	4-8 y	–	–		
	Male				
	9-13 y	–	–		
	14-18 y	–	–		
	19-30 y	–	–		
	31-50 y	–	–		
	50-70 y	–	–		
	>70 y	–	–		
	Female				
	9-13 y	–	–		
	14-18 y	–	–		
	19-30 y	–	–		
	31-50 y	–	–		
	50-70 y	–	–		
	>70 y	–	–		
	Pregnancy				
	≤18 y	–	–		
	19-30 y	–	–		
	31-50 y	–	–		
	Lactation				
	≤18 y	–	–		
	19-30 y	–	–		
	31-50 y	–	–		

12.3.7 Protein and amino acids

Function	Life stage group	RDA/AI* g/d[c]	AMDR[a]	Selected food sources	Adverse effects of excessive consumption
Serves as the major structural component of all cells in the body, and functions as enzymes, in membranes, as transport carriers, and as some hormones. During digestion and absorption dietary proteins are broken down to amino acids, which become the building blocks of these structural and functional compounds. Nine of the amino acids must be provided in the diet; these are termed indispensable amino acids. The body can make the other amino acids needed to synthesize specific structures from other amino acids	**Infants**			While no defined intake level at which potential adverse effects of protein was identified, the upper end of AMDR based on complementing the AMDR for carbohydrate and fat for the various age groups. The lower end of the AMDR is set at approximately the RDA.	While no defined intake level at which potential adverse effects of protein was identified, the upper end of AMDR based on complementing the AMDR for carbohydrate and fat for the various age groups. The lower end of the AMDR is set at approximately the RDA.
	0–6 mo	9.1*	ND[b]		
	7–12 mo	11.0	ND		
	Children				
	1–3 y	13	5–20		
	4–8 y	19	10–30		
	Male				
	9–13 y	34	10–30		
	14–18 y	52	10–30		
	19–30 y	56	10–35		
	31–50 y	56	10–35		
	50–70 y	56	10–35		
	>70 y	56	10–35		
	Female				
	9–13 y	34	10–30		
	14–18 y	46	10–30		
	19–30 y	46	10–35		
	31–50 y	46	10–35		
	50–70 y	46	10–35		
	>70 y	46	10–35		
	Pregnancy				
	≤18 y	71	10–35		
	19–30 y	71	10–35		
	31–50 y	71	10–35		
	Lactation				
	≤18 y	71	10–35		
	19–30 y	71	10–35		
	31–50 y	71	10–35		

NOTE: The tables are adapted from the DRI reports, see www.nap.edu. It represents Recommended Dietary Allowances (RDAs) in **bold type**, Adequate Intakes (AIs) in ordinary type followed by an asterisk (*). RDAs and AIs may both be used as goals for individual intake. RDAs are set to meet the needs of almost all (97 to 98 percent) individuals in a group. For healthy breastfed infants, the AI is the mean intake. The AI for other life stage and gender groups is believed to cover the needs of all individuals in the group, but lack of data prevent being able to specify with confidence the percentage of individuals covered by this intake.

a Acceptable Macronutrient Distribution Range (AMDR)[a] is the range of intake for a particular energy source that is associated with reduced risk of chronic disease while providing intakes of essential nutrients. If an individuals consumed in excess of the AMDR, there is a potential of increasing the risk of chronic diseases and insufficient intakes of essential nutrients.

b ND = Not determinable due to lack of data of adverse effects in this age group and concern with regard to lack of ability to handle excess amounts. Source of intake should be from food only to prevent high levels of intake

c Based on 1.5 g/kg/day for infants, 1.1 g/kg/day for 1-3 y, 0.95 g/kg/day for 4-13 y, 0.85 g/kg/day for 14-18 y, 0.8 g/kg/day for adults, and 1.1 g/kg/day for pregnant (using prepregnancy weight) and lactating women

12.3.8　Indispensable amino acids

Nutrient	IOM/FNB 2002 Scoring Pattern[a]	Mg/g protein	Function	Adverse effects of excessive consumption
Histidine	Histidine	18	The building blocks of all proteins in the body and some hormones. These nine amino acids must be provided in the diet and thus are termed indispensable amino acids. The body can make the other amino acids needed to synthesize specific structures from other amino acids and carbohydrate precursors.	Since there is no evidence that amino acids found in usual or even high intakes of protein from food present any risk, attention was focused on intakes of the L-form of these and other amino acid found in dietary protein and amino acid supplements. Even from well-studied amino acids, adequate dose-response data from human or animal studies on which to base a UL were not available. While no defined intake level at which potential adverse effects of protein was identified for any amino acid, this does not mean that there is no potential for adverse effects resulting from high intakes of amino acids from dietary supplements. Since data on the adverse effects of high levels of amino acid intakes from dietary supplements are limited, caution may be warranted.
Isoleucine	Isoleucine	25		
Leucine	Leucine	55		
Lysine	Lysine	51		
Methionine & Cysteine	Methionine & Cysteine	25		
Phenylalanine & Tyrosine	Phenylalanine & Tyrosine	47		
Threonine	Threonine	27		
Tryptophan	Tryptophan	7		
Valine	Valine	32		

NOTE: The table is adapted from the DRI reports, see www.nap.edu
[a] Based on the amino acid requirements derived for Preschool Children (1-3 y): (EAR for amino acid ÷ EAR for protein); for 1-3 y group where EAR for protein = 0.88 g/kg/d
→Food and Nutrition Board, Institute of Medicine, National Academies

12.4 Acceptable Macronutrient Distribution Ranges

Macronutrient	Range (percent of energy)	
	Children, 1–3 y	Children, 4–18 y
Fat	30–40	25–35
n-6 polyunsaturated fatty acids[a] (linoleic acid)	5–10	5–10
n-3 polyunsaturated fatty acids[a] (α-linolenic acid)	0.6–1.2	0.6–1.2
Carbohydrate	45–65	45–65
Protein	5–20	10–30

Macronutrients	Recommendation
Dietary cholesterol	As low as possible while consuming a nutritionally adequate diet
Trans fatty acids	As low as possible while consuming a nutritionally adequate diet
Saturated fatty acids	As low as possible while consuming a nutritionally adequate diet
Added sugars[b]	Limit to no more than 25% of total energy

a Approximately 10 percent of the total can come from longer-chain n-3 or n-6 fatty acids
b Not a recommended intake. A daily intake of added sugars that individuals should aim for to achieve a healthful diet was not set

12.5 Tolerable Upper Intake Levels

12.5.1 Vitamins

(Food and Nutrition Board, Institute of Medicine, National Academies)

Life stage group	Vitamin A (mcg/d)[a]	Vitamin C (mg/d)	Vitamin D (mcg/d)	Vitamin E (mg/d)[b,c]	Vitamin K	Thiamin	Ribo-flavin
Infants							
0–6 mo	600	ND[e]	25	ND	ND	ND	ND
6–12 mo	600	ND	38	ND	ND	ND	ND
Children							
1–3 y	600	400	63	200	ND	ND	ND
4–8 y	900	650	75	300	ND	ND	ND
Male							
9–13 y	1,700	1,200	100	600	ND	ND	ND
14–18 y	2,800	1,800	100	800	ND	ND	ND
19–30 y	3,000	2,000	100	1,000	ND	ND	ND
31–50 y	3,000	2,000	100	1,000	ND	ND	ND
51–70 y	3,000	2,000	100	1,000	ND	ND	ND
>70 y	3,000	2,000	100	1,000	ND	ND	ND
Female							
9–13 y	1,700	1,200	100	600	ND	ND	ND
14–18 y	2,800	1,800	100	800	ND	ND	ND
19–30 y	3,000	2,000	100	1,000	ND	ND	ND
31–50 y	3,000	2,000	100	1,000	ND	ND	ND
51–70 y	3,000	2,000	100	1,000	ND	ND	ND
>70 y	3,000	2,000	100	1,000	ND	ND	ND
Pregnancy							
14–18 y	2,800	1,800	100	800	ND	ND	ND
19–30 y	3,000	2,000	100	1,000	ND	ND	ND
31–50 y	3,000	2,000	100	1,000	ND	ND	ND
Lactation							
14–18 y	2,800	1,800	100	800	ND	ND	ND
19–30 y	3,000	2,000	100	1,000	ND	ND	ND
31–50 y	3,000	2,000	100	1,000	ND	ND	ND

Vitamins (cont.)								
Life stage group	Niacin (mg/d)[c]	Vitamin B_6 (mg/d)	Folate (mcg/d)[c]	Vitamin B_{12}	Panto-thenic acid	Biotin	Choline (g/d)	Carot-enoids[d]
Infants								
0-6 mo	ND	ND	ND	ND	ND	ND	ND	ND
6-12 mo	ND	ND	ND	ND	ND	ND	ND	ND
Children								
1-3 y	10	30	300	ND	ND	ND	1.0	ND
4-8 y	15	40	400	ND	ND	ND	1.0	ND
Male								
9-13 y	20	60	600	ND	ND	ND	2.0	ND
14-18 y	30	80	800	ND	ND	ND	3.0	ND
19-30 y	35	100	1,000	ND	ND	ND	3.5	ND
31-50 y	35	100	1,000	ND	ND	ND	3.5	ND
51-70 y	35	100	1,000	ND	ND	ND	3.5	ND
>70 y	35	100	1,000	ND	ND	ND	3.5	ND
Female								
9-13 y	20	60	600	ND	ND	ND	2.0	ND
14-18 y	30	80	800	ND	ND	ND	3.0	ND
19-30 y	35	100	1,000	ND	ND	ND	3.5	ND
31-50 y	35	100	1,000	ND	ND	ND	3.5	ND
51-70 y	35	100	1,000	ND	ND	ND	3.5	ND
>70 y	35	100	1,000	ND	ND	ND	3.5	ND
Pregnancy								
14-18 y	30	80	800	ND	ND	ND	3.0	ND
19-30 y	35	100	1,000	ND	ND	ND	3.5	ND
31-50 y	35	100	1,000	ND	ND	ND	3.5	ND
Lactation								
14-18 y	30	80	800	ND	ND	ND	3.0	ND
19-30 y	35	100	1,000	ND	ND	ND	3.5	ND
31-50 y	35	100	1,000	ND	ND	ND	3.5	ND

NOTE: A Tolerable Upper Intake Level (UL) is the highest level of daily nutrient intake that is likely to pose no risk of adverse health effects to almost all individuals in the general population. Unless otherwise specified, the UL represents total intake from food, water, and supplements. Due to a lack of suitable data, ULs could not be established for vitamin K, thiamin, riboflavin, vitamin B12, pantothenic acid, biotin, and carotenoids. In the absence of a UL, extra caution may be warranted in consuming levels above recommended intakes. Members of the general population should be advised not to routinely exceed the UL. The UL is not meant to apply to individuals who are treated with the nutrient under medical supervision or to individuals with predisposing conditions that modify their sensitivity to the nutrient.

[a] As preformed vitamin A only

[b] As α-tocopherol; applies to any form of supplemental α-tocopherol

[c] The ULs for vitamin E, niacin, and folate apply to synthetic forms obtained from supplements, fortified foods, or a combination of the two

[d] ß-Carotene supplements are advised only to serve as a provitamin A source for individuals at risk of vitamin A deficiency

[e] ND = Not determinable due to lack of data of adverse effects in this age group and concern with regard to lack of ability to handle excess amounts. Source of intake should be from food only to prevent high levels of intake.

12.5.2	Elements								
Life stage group	Arsenic[a]	Boron (mg/d)	Calcium (mg/d)	Chromium	Copper (mcg/d)	Fluoride (mg/d)	Iodine (mcg/d)	Iron (mg/d)	Magnesium (mg/d)[b]
Infants									
0-6 mo	ND[c]	ND	1,000	ND	ND	0.7	ND	40	ND
6-12 mo	ND	ND	1,500	ND	ND	0.9	ND	40	ND
Children									
1-3 y	ND	3	2,500	ND	1,000	1.3	200	40	65
4-8 y	ND	6	2,500	ND	3,000	2.2	300	40	110
Male									
9-13 y	ND	11	3,000	ND	5,000	10	600	40	350
14-18 y	ND	17	3,000	ND	8,000	10	900	45	350
19-30 y	ND	20	2,500	ND	10,000	10	1,100	45	350
31-50 y	ND	20	2,500	ND	10,000	10	1,100	45	350
51-70 y	ND	20	2,000	ND	10,000	10	1,100	45	350
>70 y	ND	20	2,000	ND	10,000	10	1,100	45	350
Female									
9-13 y	ND	11	3,000	ND	5,000	10	600	40	350
14-18 y	ND	17	3,000	ND	8,000	10	900	45	350
19-30 y	ND	20	2,500	ND	10,000	10	1,100	45	350
31-50 y	ND	20	2,500	ND	10,000	10	1,100	45	350
51-70 y	ND	20	2,000	ND	10,000	10	1,100	45	350
>70 y	ND	20	2,000	ND	10,000	10	1,100	45	350
Pregnancy									
14-18 y	ND	17	3,000	ND	8,000	10	900	45	350
19-30 y	ND	20	2,500	ND	10,000	10	1,100	45	350
31-50 y	ND	20	2,500	ND	10,000	10	1,100	45	350
Lactation									
14-18 y	ND	17	3,000	ND	8,000	10	900	45	350
19-30 y	ND	20	2,500	ND	10,000	10	1,100	45	350
31-50 y	ND	20	2,500	ND	10,000	10	1,100	45	350

Elements (cont.)										
Life stage group	Manganese (mg/d)	Molybdenum (mcg/d)	Nickel (mg/d)	Phosphorus (g/d)	Selenium (mcg/d)	Silicon[c]	Vanadium (mg/d)[d]	Zinc (mg/d)	Sodium (g/d)	Chloride (g/d)
Infants										
0–6 mo	ND	ND	ND	ND	45	ND	ND	4	ND	ND
6–12 mo	ND	ND	ND	ND	60	ND	ND	5	ND	ND
Children										
1–3 y	2	300	0.2	3	90	ND	ND	7	1.5	2.3
4–8 y	3	600	0.3	3	150	ND	ND	12	1.9	2.9
Male										
9–13 y	6	1,100	0.6	4	280	ND	ND	23	2.2	3.4
14–18 y	9	1,700	1.0	4	400	ND	ND	34	2.3	3.6
19–30 y	11	2,000	1.0	4	400	ND	1.8	40	2.3	3.6
31–50 y	11	2,000	1.0	4	400	ND	1.8	40	2.3	3.6
51–70 y	11	2,000	1.0	4	400	ND	1.8	40	2.3	3.6
>70 y	11	2,000	1.0	3	400	ND	1.8	40	2.3	3.6
Female										
9–13 y	6	1,100	0.6	4	280	ND	ND	23	2.2	3.4
14–18 y	9	1,700	1.0	4	400	ND	ND	34	2.3	3.6
19–30 y	11	2,000	1.0	4	400	ND	1.8	40	2.3	3.6
31–50 y	11	2,000	1.0	4	400	ND	1.8	40	2.3	3.6
51–70 y	11	2,000	1.0	4	400	ND	1.8	40	2.3	3.6
>70 y	11	2,000	1.0	3	400	ND	1.8	40	2.3	3.6
Pregnancy										
14–18 y	9	1,700	1.0	3.5	400	ND	ND	34	2.3	3.6
19–30 y	11	2,000	1.0	3.5	400	ND	ND	40	2.3	3.6
31–50 y	11	2,000	1.0	3.5	400	ND	ND	40	2.3	3.6
Lactation										
14–18 y	9	1,700	1.0	4	400	ND	ND	34	2.3	3.6
19–30 y	11	2,000	1.0	4	400	ND	ND	40	2.3	3.6
31–50 y	11	2,000	1.0	4	400	ND	ND	40	2.3	3.6

NOTE: A Tolerable Upper Intake Level (UL) is the highest level of daily nutrient intake that is likely to pose no risk of adverse health effects to almost all individuals in the general population. Unless otherwise specified, the UL represents total intake from food, water, and supplements. Due to a lack of suitable data, ULs could not be established for vitamin K, thiamin, riboflavin, vitamin B12, pantothenic acid, biotin, and carotenoids. In the absence of a UL, extra caution may be warranted in consuming levels above recommended intakes. Members of the general population should be advised not to routinely exceed the UL. The UL is not meant to apply to individuals who are treated with the nutrient under medical supervision or to individuals with predisposing conditions that modify their sensitivity to the nutrient.

[a] Although the UL was not determined for arsenic, there is no justification for adding arsenic to food or supplements

[b] The ULs for magnesium represent intake from a pharmacological agent only and do not include intake from food and water

[c] Although silicon has not been shown to cause adverse effects in humans, there is no justification for adding silicon to supplements

[d] Although vanadium in food has not been shown to cause adverse effects in humans, there is no justification for adding vanadium to food and vanadium supplements should be used with caution. The UL is based on adverse effects in laboratory animals and this data could be used to set a UL for adults but not children and adolescents

[e] ND = Not determinable due to lack of data of adverse effects in this age group and concern with regard to lack of ability to handle excess amounts. Source of intake should be from food only to prevent high levels of intake

12.6 Electrolytes and Water Nutrient

12.6.1 Sodium

Function	Life stage group	AI (g/d)	ULa (g/d)	Selected food sources	Adverse effects of excessive consumption	Special considerations
Maintains fluid volume outside of cells and thus normal cell function	**Infants**			Processed foods to which sodium chloride (salt)/ benzoate/ phosphate have been added; salted meats, nuts, cold cuts; margarine; butter; salt added to foods in cooking or at the table. Salt is ~ 40% sodium by weight	Hypertension; increased risk of cardiovascular disease and stroke	The AI is set based on being able to obtain a nutritionally adequate diet for other nutrients and to meet the needs for sweat losses for individuals engaged in recommended levels of physical activity. Individuals engaged in activity at higher levels or in humid climates resulting in excessive sweat may need more than the AI. The UL applies to apparently healthy individuals without hypertension; it thus may be too high for individuals who already have hypertension or who are under the care of a health care professional.
	0–6 mo	0.12	NDb			
	7–12 mo	0.37	NDb			
	Children					
	1–3 y	1.0	1.5			
	4–8 y	1.2	1.9			
	Male					
	9–13 y	1.5	2.2			
	14–18 y	1.5	2.3			
	19–30 y	1.5	2.3			
	31–50 y	1.5	2.3			
	50–70 y	1.3	2.3			
	> 70 y	1.2	2.3			
	Female					
	9–13 y	1.5	2.2			
	14–18 y	1.5	2.3			
	19–30 y	1.5	2.3			
	31–50 y	1.5	2.3			
	50–70 y	1.3	2.3			
	> 70 y	1.2	2.3			
	Pregnancy					
	14–18 y	1.5	2.3			
	19–50 y	1.5	2.3			
	Lactation					
	14–18 y	1.5	2.3			
	19–50 y	1.5	2.3			

12.6.2 Chloride

Function	Life stage group	AI (g/d)	UL[a] (g/d)	Selected food sources	Adverse effects of excessive consumption	Special considerations
With sodium, maintains fluid volume outside of cells and thus normal cell function	**Infants**			See above; about 60% by weight of salt	In concert with sodium, results in hypertension	Chloride is lost usually with sodium in sweat, as well as in vomiting and diarrhea. The AI and UL are equimolar in amount to sodium since most of sodium in diet comes as sodium chloride (salt).
	0-6 mo	0.18	ND[b]			
	7-12 mo	0.57	ND[b]			
	Children					
	1-3 y	1.5	2.3			
	4-8 y	1.9	2.9			
	Male					
	9-13 y	2.3	3.4			
	14-18 y	2.3	3.6			
	19-30 y	2.3	3.6			
	31-50 y	2.3	3.6			
	50-70 y	2.0	3.6			
	> 70 y	1.8	3.6			
	Female					
	9-13 y	2.3	3.4			
	14-18 y	2.3	3.6			
	19-30 y	2.3	3.6			
	31-50 y	2.3	3.6			
	50-70 y	2.0	3.6			
	> 70 y	1.8	3.6			
	Pregnancy					
	14-18 y	2.3	3.6			
	19-50 y	2.3	3.6			
	Lactation					
	14-18 y	2.3	3.6			
	19-50 y	2.3	3.6			

12.6.3 Potassium

Function	Life stage group	AI (g/d)	UL[a] No UL.	Selected food sources	Adverse effects of excessive consumption	Special considerations
Maintains fluid volume inside/outside of cells and thus normal cell function; acts to blunt the rise of blood pressure in response to excess sodium intake, and decrease markers of bone turnover and recurrence of kidney stones	**Infants**			Fruits and vegetables; dried peas; dairy products; meats, and nuts	None documented from food alone; however, potassium from supplements or salt substitutes can result in hyperkalemia and possibly sudden death if excess is consumed by individuals with chronic renal insufficiency (kidney disease) or diabetes	Individuals taking drugs for cardiovascular disease such as ACE inhibitors, ARBs (Angiontensin Receptor Blockers), or potassium sparing diuretics should be careful to not consume supplements containing potassium and may need to consume less than the AI for potassium
	0–6 mo	0.4	–			
	7–12 mo	0.7	–			
	Children					
	1–3 y	3.0	–			
	4–8 y	3.8	–			
	Male					
	9–13 y	4.5	–			
	14–18 y	4.7	–			
	19–30 y	4.7	–			
	31–50 y	4.7	–			
	50–70 y	4.7	–			
	> 70 y	4.7	–			
	Female					
	9–13 y	4.5	–			
	14–18 y	4.7	–			
	19–30 y	4.7	–			
	31–50 y	4.7	–			
	50–70 y	4.7	–			
	> 70 y	4.7	–			
	Pregnancy					
	14–18 y	4.7	–			
	19–50 y	4.7	–			
	Lactation					
	14–18 y	5.1	–			
	19–50 y	5.1	–			

12.6.4 Water

Function	Life stage group	AI (g/d)	ULa No UL.	Selected food sources	Adverse effects of excessive consumption	Special considerations
Maintains homeostasis in the body and allows for transport of nutrients to cells and removal and excretion of waste products of metabolism	**Infants**			All beverages, including water, as well as moisture in foods (high moisture foods include watermelon, meats, soups, etc.)	No UL because normally functioning kidneys can handle more than 0.7 L (24 oz) of fluid per hour; symptoms of water intoxication include hyponatremia which can result in heart failure and rhabdomyolysis (skeletal muscle tissue injury) which can lead to kidney failure	Recommended intakes for water are based on median intakes of generally healthy individuals who are adequately hydrated; individuals can be adequately hydrated at levels below as well as above the AIs provided. The AIs provided are for total water in temperate climates. All sources can contribute to total water needs: beverages (including tea, coffee, juices, sodas, and drinking water) and moisture found in foods. Moisture in food accounts for about 20% of total water intake. Thirst and consumption of beverages at meals are adequate to maintain hydration.
	0–6 mo	0.7	–			
	7–12 mo	0.8	–			
	Children					
	1–3 y	1.3	–			
	4–8 y	1.7	–			
	Male					
	9–13 y	2.4	–			
	14–18 y	3.3	–			
	19–30 y	3.7	–			
	31–50 y	3.7	–			
	50–70 y	3.7	–			
	> 70 y	3.7	–			
	Female					
	9–13 y	2.1	–			
	14–18 y	2.3	–			
	19–30 y	2.7	–			
	31–50 y	2.7	–			
	50–70 y	2.7	–			
	> 70 y	2.7	–			
	Pregnancy					
	14–18 y	3.0	–			
	19–50 y	3.0	–			
	Lactation					
	14–18 y	3.8	–			
	19–50 y	3.8	–			

12.6.5 Inorganic sulfate

Function	Life stage group	AI (g/d)	UL[a] No UL.	Selected food sources	Adverse effects of excessive consumption	Special considerations
Required for biosynthesis of 3'-phospho-adenosine-5'-phosphate (PAPS), which provides sulfate when sulfur-containing compounds are needed such as chondroitin sulfate and cerebroside sulfate	**Infants**	No recommended intake was set as adequate sulfate is available from dietary inorganic sulfate from water and foods, and from sources of organic sulfate, such as glutathione and the sulfur amino acids methionine and cysteine. Metabolic breakdown of the recommended intake for protein and sulfur amino acids should provide adequate inorganic sulfate for synthesis of required sulfur-containing compounds	–	Dried fruit (dates, raisins, dried apples), soy flour, fruit juices, coconut milk, red and white wine, bread, as well as meats that are high in sulfur amino acids	Osmotic diarrhea was observed in areas where water supply had high levels; odor and off taste usually limit intake, and thus no UL was set	–
	0–6 mo					
	7–12 mo					
	Children					
	1–3 y					
	4–8 y					
	Male					
	9–13 y					
	14–18 y					
	19–30 y					
	31–50 y					
	50–70 y					
	> 70 y					
	Female					
	9–13 y					
	14–18 y					
	19–30 y					
	31–50 y					
	50–70 y					
	> 70 y					
	Pregnancy					
	14–18 y					
	19–50 y					
	Lactation					
	14–18 y					
	19–50 y					

NOTE: The table is adapted from the DRI reports. See www.nap.edu. Adequate Intakes (AIs) may be used as a goal for individual intake. For healthy breastfed infants, the AI is the mean intake. The AI for other life stage and gender groups is believed to cover the needs of all individuals in the group, but lack of data prevent being able to specify with confidence the percentage of individuals covered by this intake; therefore, no Recommended Dietary Allowance (RDA) was set.

[a] UL = The maximum level of daily nutrient intake that is likely to pose no risk of adverse effects. Unless otherwise specified, the UL represents total intake from food, water, and supplements. Due to lack of suitable data, ULs could not be established for potassium, water, and inorganic sulfate. In the absence of ULs, extra caution may be warranted in consuming levels above recommended intakes.

[b] ND = Not determinable due to lack of data of adverse effects in this age group and concern with regard to lack of ability to handle excess amounts. Source of intake should be from food only to prevent high levels of intake.

List of references

[103] Dietary Reference Intakes for Calcium, Phosphorous, Magnesium, Vitamin D, and Fluoride (1997); Dietary Reference Intakes for Thiamin, Riboflavin, Niacin, Vitamin B6, Folate, Vitamin B12, Pantothenic Acid, Biotin, and Choline (1998); Dietary Reference Intakes for Vitamin C, Vitamin E, Selenium, and Carotenoids (2000); Dietary Reference Intakes for Vitamin A, Vitamin K, Arsenic, Boron, Chromium, Copper, Iodine, Iron, Manganese, Molybdenum, Nickel, Silicon, Vanadium, and Zinc (2001); Dietary Reference Intakes for Water, Potassium, Sodium, Chloride, and Sulfate (2005); and Dietary Reference Intakes for Calcium and Vitamin D (2011). These reports may be accessed via www.nap.edu.

13 Appendix

13.1 High Oxalate Foods

High oxalate foods	
Vegetables	Beets, celery, collard greens, eggplant, escarole, leeks, okra, parsley, rhubarb, rutabagas, spinach, sweet potatoes, swiss chard
Fruit	Blackberries, blueberries, concord grapes, currants, figs, gooseberries
Beverages	Dark beer, ovaltine, tea (black)
Nuts	Almonds, hazelnuts, peanuts, pecans
Legumes	Lentils, soybeans
Miscellaneous	Chocolate, cocoa, grits, white corn, wheat germ

13.2 Nutrient–Drug Interactions

(see reference [104])

13.2.1 General concepts
- Nutrients and drugs (prescription and over-the-counter) can reciprocally affect each other's absorption, pharmacokinetics, and action
- Consequences include nutritional deficiencies/toxicities and drug effectiveness/toxicities

13.2.2 Specific interactions drugs have on nutrients
- Appetite:
  - Increased: mirtazapine, amitriptyline, cyproheptadine, haloperidol, risperidone, quetiapine, carvedilol, propranolol, clonidine, glucocorticoids, megestrol acetate, medroxyprogesterone acetate, testosterone, sulfonylureas
  - Decreased: phentermine, diethylpropion, amphetamines, methylphenidate, bupropion, venlafaxine
- Altered taste:
  - Bitter: aspirin, carbamazepine, 5FU, isosorbide, levodopa, Risperdal
  - Metallic: allopurinol, captopril, lithium, metformin, metronidazole, sulphasalazine, nifedipine

Specific interactions drugs have on nutrients (cont.)

- Decreased intake due to GI symptoms (nausea, vomiting, diarrhea, abdominal discomfort, stomatitis/mucositis, xerostomia):
  - Chemotherapy
  - Laxatives
  - Antibiotics
  - Opioids/opiates
  - Antidepressants
- Impaired nutrient absorption:
  - Aluminum hydroxide-phosphate
  - Phenytoin: folate
  - Cholestyramine: fat-soluble vitamins (A, D, E, K)
  - Tetracycline: calcium, iron, magnesium, zinc
  - H2-blockers: vitamin B12
  - Methotrexate: folate, vitamin B12
- Impaired nutrient production
  - Cephalosporins: vitamin K from intestinal bacteria
- Impaired nutrient metabolism
  - Oral contraceptives: pyridoxine and folate
- ↑ nutrient excretion
  - Furosemide: thiamine, potassium, magnesium, calcium
  - Aspirin: folate, iron (indirectly with gastric bleed)
  - Phenytoin: vitamin D

13.2.3 Specific interactions nutrients have on drugs

- Impaired drug absorption:
  - Food many drugs require an empty stomach to facilitate absorption (eg, antibiotics, digitalis, captopril, sucralfate)
  - Acidic foods inactivate or dissolve certain medications (enterically coated tablets)
  - Dairy tetracycline
  - Calcium, iron tetracycline, levothyroxine
  - Soy protein levothyroxine
  - High protein methyldopa
- Altered drug metabolism:
  - Aged/fermented foods have tyramine which interacts with monoamine oxidase inhibitors and can cause hypertension
  - Vitamin K impairs anti-coagulant activity
  - Indolic compounds (broccoli, cabbage, cauliflower) increases drug metabolism
  - Grapefruit inhibits cytochrome p450 and intestinal transport proteins

Specific interactions nutrients have on drugs (cont.)

- Drug excretion:
  - Absence of certain nutrients (protein, carbohydrate, fat) impairs hepatic drug metabolism
  - Vitamin C ↑ urinary acidity and ↓ excretion of aspirin
- Increased adverse effects
- Alcohol metformin (increases lactate production)

13.3   ICD-9 & ICD-10 Codes

13.3.1   Nutritional diagnoses

Diagnosis	ICD-9	ICD-10 (October 2014)
Cachexia	799.4	C80.9
Mild PEM	263.1	E44.1
Moderate PEM	263.0	E44
Severe PEM	262.0	E43
Unspecified PEM	263.9	E46
Kwashiorkor	260	E40
Nutritional marasmus	261	E41
Marasmic kwashiorkor	260	E42
Malnutrition following GI surgery	579.3	K91.2

13.3.2   Gastrointestinal diagnoses

Diagnosis	ICD-9	ICD-10 (October 2014)
Celiac disease	579.0	K90.0
Crohn's disease	555.9	K50.9
Dysphagia	787.2	R13
Fistula of intestine	569.81	K63.2
Gastrointestinal hemorrhage	578.9	K92.2
Gastroparesis	536.3	K31.8
Ileus	560.1	K56.7
Intestinal malabsorption	579.9	K90.9
Intestinal obstruction	560.9	K56.6

Diagnosis	ICD-9	ICD-10 (October 2014)
Irritable bowel syndrome	564.1	K58.0
Ischemic bowel disease	557.9	K55.9
Post surgical malabsorption	564.4	K91.2
Ulcerative colitis	556.9	K51.9
Vomiting after GI surgery	564.3	K91.0

13.3.3 Macronutrient deficiencies

Diagnosis	ICD-9	ICD-10 (October 2014)
Protein losing enteropathy	579.8	K90.89
Hypoalbuminemia	273.8	E88.09
Essential fatty acid deficiency	277.85	E63.0

13.3.4 Electrolyte abnormalities

Diagnosis	ICD-9	ICD-10 (October 2014)
Hypercalcemia	275.42	E83.5
Hypocalcemia	275.41	E83.5
Hyperkalemia	276.7	E87.5
Hypokalemia	276.8	E87.6
Hypernatremia	276.0	E87.0
Hyponatremia	276.1	E87.1
Hypermagnesemia	275.2	E83.41
Hypomagnesemia	275.2	E83.41

13.3.5 Micronutrient deficiencies

Diagnosis	ICD-9	ICD-10 (October 2014)
Vitamin A deficiency	264	E50
Thiamine deficiency	265.1	E51
Riboflavin deficiency	266.0	E530
Niacin deficiency	265.2	E52
Pyridoxine deficiency	266.1	E531

Diagnosis	ICD-9	ICD-10 (October 2014)
Vitamin B12 deficiency	266.2	E53.8
Ascorbic acid deficiency	267	E54
Vitamin D deficiency	268.0	E55
Dietary calcium deficiency	269.3	E58
Iron deficiency	280.0	E611
Chromium deficiency	269.3	E614
Selenium deficiency	269.3	E59
Zinc deficiency	269.3	E60

13.3.6 Miscellaneous

Diagnosis	ICD-9	ICD-10 (October 2014)
Catheter related bloodstream infection	999.31	T80.211
Cheilitis	528.5	K13.0
Chylous pleural effusion	511.89	J94.0
Chylous ascites	457.8	I89.8
Glossitis	529.0	K14.0
Morbid obesity	278.01	E66.01
Obesity	278.0	E66
Sequelae of hyperalimenatation	999	E68
Sequelae of malnutrition and other nutritional deficiencies	X	E64
Stress hyperglycemia	790.29	R73.9

13.4 Medicare Guidelines for Home TPN

Medicare guidelines: Parenteral and enteral nutrition

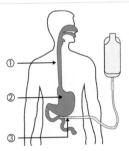
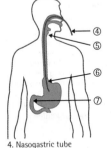

1. Esophagus
2. Stomach
3. Jejunostomy feeding tube

4. Nasogastric tube
5. Pharynx
6. Cardiac sphincter
7. Pyloric sphincter

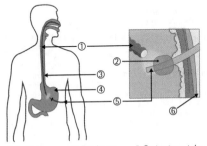

1. Endoscope
2. Balloon
3. Esophagus
4. Stomach
5. Gastrostomy tube
6. Skin

13.4.1 Total parenteral nutrition

Parenteral nutrition is covered for patients with permanent, severe disease of the gastro-intestinal tract that prevents absorption of sufficient nutrients to maintain weight and strength commensurate with the patient's overall health status

Basic criteria

A patient must meet two basic criteria:

- **Permanence**: Permanence is determined if, in the judgment of the attending physician and substantiated in the medical record, the condition is of long and indefinite duration (ordinarily at least 3 months)
- **Malabsorption of nutrients:** The patient must have
  - Condition involving the small intestine and/or its exocrine glands which significantly impairs the absorption of nutrients, OR
  - (Disease of the stomach and/or intestine which is a motility disorder and impairs the ability of nutrients to be transported through the GI system

Additional documentation

It is required to support the medical necessity when the following conditions occur:

- Total daily intake is <20 kcal/kg or >35 kcal/kg
- Protein is <0.8 and >1.5 gm/kg/day
- Dextrose concentration is <10%
- There are >15 units of lipids per month (20%) (1 unit 500 mL) or 30 units of 10%/month
- TPN infusion occurs <7 days/week
- There is a need for special nutrients (ie, renal, hepatic formulas)

13.4.2 Coverage information

Covered TPN

- The patient has undergone recent (within the past 3 months) massive small bowel resection leaving ≤5 feet of small bowel beyond the ligament of Treitz
- The patient has a short bowel syndrome that is severe enough that the patient has net gastrointestinal fluid and electrolyte malabsorption such that, on an oral intake of 2.5–3 liters/day, the enteral losses exceed 50% of the oral/enteral intake and the urine output is <1 liter/day
- The patient requires bowel rest for at least 3 months and is intravenously receiving 20–35 kcal/kg/day for treatment of symptomatic pancreatitis with/without pancreatic pseudocyst, severe exacerbation of regional enteritis, or a proximal enterocutaneous fistula where tube feeding distal to the fistula isn't possible.

Covered TPN (cont.)

- The patient has complete mechanical small bowel obstruction where surgery is not an option
- The patient is significantly malnourished (10% weight loss over 3 months or less and serum albumin ≤3.4 g/dL) and has very severe fat malabsorption (fecal fat exceeds 50% of oral/enteral intake on a diet of at least 50 gm of fat/day as measured by a standard 72 hours fecal fat test)
- The patient is significantly malnourished (10% weight loss over 3 months or less and serum albumin ≤3.4 g/dL) and has a severe motility disturbance of the small intestine and/or stomach which is unresponsive to prokinetic medication and is demonstrated either:
  – Scintigraphically (solid meal gastric emptying study demonstrates that the isotope fails to reach the right colon by 6 hours following ingestion) or
  – Radiographically (barium or radiopaque pellets fail to reach the right colon by 6 hours following administration). These studies must be performed when the patient is nor acutely ill and is not on any medication which would decrease bowel motility
- Unresponsiveness to prokinetic medication is defined as the presence of daily symptoms of nausea and vomiting while taking maximal doses
- The patient is malnourished (10% weight loss over 3 months or less and serum albumin ≤3.4 g/dL) and a disease and clinical condition has been documented as being present and it has nor responded to altering the manner of delivery of appropriate nutrients (eg, slow infusion of nutrients through a rube with tip located in the stomach or jejunum)

May be covered with failed tube feeding trial

- Moderate fat malabsorption fecal fat exceeds 25% of oral/enteral intake on a diet of at least 50 g of fat/day as measured by a standard 72 hours fecal fat rest
- Diagnosis of malabsorption with objective confirmation by methods other than 72 hours fecal fat test (eg, Sudan stain of stool, d-xylose test, etc)
- Gastroparesis which has been demonstrated:
  – Radiographically or scintigraphically as described in criteria F with the isotopes or pellets failing to reach the jejunum in 3-6 hours, OR
  – By manometric motility studies with results consistent with an abnormal gastric emptying, and which is unresponsive to prokinetic medication
- Small bowel motility disturbance which is unresponsive to prokinetic medication, demonstrated with a gastric to right colon transit time between 3-6 hours

May be covered with failed tube feeding trial (cont.)

- Small bowel resection leaving >5 feet of small bowel beyond the ligament of Treitz
- Short bowel syndrome which is not severe (as defined by criteria B). See actual Medicare guidelines
- Mild to moderate exacerbation of regional enteritis, or an enterocutaneous fistula
- Partial mechanical small bowel obstruction where surgery is not an option

Not covered

- Swallowing disorder
- Temporary defect in gastric emptying such as a metabolic or electrolyte disorder
- Psychological disorder impairing food intake such as depression
- Metabolic disorder inducing anorexia such as cancer
- Physical disorder impairing food intake such as the dyspnea of severe pulmonary or cardiac disease
- Side effect of a medication
- Renal failure and/or dialysis

List of references

[104] Van Zyl. S Afr J Clin Nutr 2011; 24: S38–S41

3.5 Abbreviations

→	leads to, causes
↑	increased, elevated
↓	decreased, depressed
40C/ 30P/30F	40% carbohydrate/ 30% protein/ 30% fat
F	degree Fahrenheit
α	alpha
α-MSH	alpha-melanocyte stimulating hormone
A	age (yrs)
AA	amino acids
A1c	hemoglobin A1c
AACE	American Association of Clinical Endocrinologists
ABC	ATP-binding cassette
ACE	angiotensin converting enzyme
ACI	acute critical illness
ACP	acyl carrier protein
ACS	American College of Surgeons
ACTH	Adrenocorticotropic hormone
ADA	American Diabetes Association
ADH	antidiuretic hormone
AE	adverse effects
AFP	Alpha-fetoprotein
AGA	American Gastroenterological Association
AGB	adjustable gastric band
AGRP	agouti related peptide
AHA	American Heart Association
AI	adequate intake

AIDS	acquired immune deficiency syndrome
ALT	alanine transaminase
AMDR	adequate/acceptable macro-nutrient distribution range
ANA	antinuclear antibodies
approx	approximately
ARDS	acute respiratory distress syndrome
Arg	arginine
ASMBS	American Society for Metabolic and Bariatric Surgery
ASPEN	American Society for Parenteral and Enteral Nutrition
AST	Aspartate Aminotransferase
ATP	adenosine triphosphate
B	burn
β	beta
BCAA	branched chain amino acids
BG	blood glucose
BIA	bioelectrical impedance
BID	twice a day
BIPAP	bilevel positive airway pressure
BMI	body mass index
BMR	basal metabolic rate
BMT	bone marrow transplant
BNP	brain natriuretic peptide
BP	blood pressure
BPD	biliopancreatic diversion

BPDDS	biliopancreatic diversion with duodenal switch
BUN	blood urea nitrogen
BV	biological value
Ca	calcium
CA	cancer antigen
CAD	coronary artery disease
CAMP	Christie, Atkins, and Munch-Peterson
CART	cocaine, and amphetamine-related transcript
CBC	complete blood count
cc	cubic centimeter
CCI	chronic critical illness
CCK	cholecystokinin
CD	Cluster of differentiation
CFTR	cystic fibrosis transmembrane conductance regulator
CHF	congestive heart failure
CI	contraindication(s)
CKD	chronic kidney disease
Cl	chlorine
CL	class
CHO	carbohydrate
CK	creatine kinase
cm	centimeter
CMS	Centers for Medicare and Medicaid Services
CO_2	carbon dioxide
cont.	continue
CPAP	continuous positive airway pressure
CPG	clinical practice guidelines

CPR	c-reactive protein
Cr	chromium
CT	computerized tomography
CTx	c-telopeptide
cu	copper
CVD	cardiovascular disease
CVVH	continuous veno-venous hemofiltration
d	day
D5W	dextrose 5% in water
DASH	dietary approaches to stop hypertension
DDX	differential diagnosis
DFE	dietary folate equivalents
DGA	Dietary Guidelines for Americans
DHEA	dehydroepiandrosterone
DO	dosing
DHA	docosahexaenoic acid
DJB	duodenojejunal bypass
DM	diabetes mellitus
DMT1	divalent metal transporter-1
DNA	deoxyribonucleic acid
DPP-4	dipeptidyl peptidase-4
DRG	diagnosis related groups
DRIs	dietary reference intakes
DS	dietary Supplements
DSHEA	dietary supplement health and education act
DVT	deep venous thrombosis
DXA	dual x-ray absorptiometry

EAR	estimated average requirement		GERD	gastroesophageal reflux disease
EBW	excess body weight		GH	growth hormone
EDTA	ethylenediaminetetraacetic acid		GI	gastrointestinal
			GI	glycemic index
EE	energy expenditure		GIP	glucose-dependent insulinotropic peptide
EF	effects			
EFA	essential fatty acids		GLA	gamma linoleic acid
eg,	for example (latin: exempli gratia)		Gln	glutamine
			GLP1	glucagon-like peptide-1
EHL	elimination half life		GRV	gastric residual volume
EKG	electrocardiogram		GVHD	graft vs host disease
EN	enteral nutrition		h	hours
EPA	eicosapentaenoic acid		H	halal
ESRD	end stage renal disease		HBDH	Hydroxybutyrate dehydroge- nase
F	female			
FAD	component of flavin adenine dinucleotide		HD	hemodialysis
			HDL	high density lipoprotein
FBG	fasting blood glucose		HGH	human growth hormone
FGF23	fibroblast growth factor 23		HIV	human immunodeficiency virus
FMN	flavin mononucleotide			
FNB	food and nutrition board		HR	heart rate
FOS	fructooligosaccharide (prebiotic fibers)		hSMVT	human sodium dependent multivitamin transporter
			Ht	height
FPIES	food protein induced enterocolitis syndrome		HTN	hypertension
			I	iodine
FSH	follicle stimulating hormone		IBD	inflammatory bowel disease
G	gluten-free/ gender		lbs	pounds
G6PD	glucose-6-phosphate dehydrogenase		IBS	irritable bowel syndrome
			IBW	ideal body weight
g/gm	gram		ICD	international classification of diseases

ICU	intensive care unit		LCFA	long chain fatty acids
IDPN	intradialytic parenteral nutrition		LCT	long chain triglyceride
IGF	Insulin-like Growth Factor		LDH	lactate dehydrogenase
IL-4	interleukin-4		LDL	low density lipoprotein
in	inches		LES	lower esophageal sphincter
Info	information		LFT	liver function tests
IJEE	ireton jones energy equations		LH	luteinizing hormone
INA	immune neuroendocrine axis		LOS	length of stay
INR	international normalized ratio		LRYGB	laparoscopic Roux-en-Y gastric
IOM	institute of medicine		m	meter
IU	international unit		M	male
IV	intravenous		MA	mechanism of action
J tube	jejunostomy tube		MAO	monoamine oxidase
JIB	jejunal-ileal bypass		MCA	Mucin like antigen
K	kosher		MCT	medium chain triglyceride
K	potassium		MDH	malate dehydrogenase
kcal	kilocalories		MEE	measured energy expenditure
KCl	potassium chloride		MEN	multiple endocrine neoplasms
kg	kilogram		mEq	milliequivalent
KVO	keep vein open		Mg	magnesium
L	liter		mg	miligram
L	lactose-free		min	minute
Lact	lactation risk category		ml	milliliter
LAGB	laparoscopic adjustable gastric band		Mn	manganese
LAP	leukocyte alkaline phosphatase		MNT	medical nutrition therapy
LASA	lipid-associated sialic acid		mo	months
LBPDDS	laparoscopic biliopancreatic diversion with duodenal switch		mOsmol/g	milliosmoles per gram
			MRI	magnetic resonance imaging
			MRP	multidrug resistance associated protein

MRSA	Methicillin resistant Staphylococcus aureus	NOTES	natural orifice transluminal endoscopic surgery
MS	mental status	NPO	nil per os, nothing by mouth
MSH	melanocyte stimulating hormone	NPY	neuropeptide Y
MSPI	milk soy protein intolerance	NRI	nutritional risk index
MTE	multiple trace elements	NRS	nutritional risk screening
MUFA	monounsaturated fatty acids	NS	normal saline
MUST	malnutrition universal screening tool	NSAID	non steroidal anti-inflammatory drug
MVI	multivitamins	NTx	N-telopeptide
N	nitrogen	O	oral/obesity
Na	sodium	OBPDDS	open biliopancreatic diversion with duodenal switch
N/A	not applicable	OHS	obesity hypoventilation syndrome
NADH	nicotinamide adenine dinucleotide	ORYGB	open Roux-en-Y gastric bypass
NAFLD	non alcoholic fatty liver disease	OSA	obstructive sleep apnea
NASH	nonalcoholic steatohepatitis	oz	ounce
NCD	national coverage decision	[P]	plasma
NCEP	national cholesterol education program	P5P	pyridoxal-5'-phosphate
ND	not determinable	PACI	prolonged acute critical illness
NE	niacin equivalents	PCA	patient controlled analgesia
NGT/ NG tube	nasogastric tube	PCFT	protein coupled folate transporter
NHLBI	National heart, Lung, and Blood Institute	PCOS	polycystic ovary syndrome
		PD	peritoneal dialysis
NIPHS	non-insulinoma pancreatogenous hypoglycemia syndrome	PEG	percutaneous gastrostomy
		PEM	protein energy malnutrition
NKF-K/ DOQI	National Kidney Foundation's Kidney Disease Outcomes Quality Initiative	PEP	protein energy provision
		PET	positron emission tomography
		pH	potential of hydrogen
		Phos	phosphorus

PICC	peripherally-inserted central catheter
PN	parenteral nutrition
POD	postoperative day
POMC	proopiomelanocortin
PPN	peripheral parenteral nutrition
PRC	pregnancy risk category
PSA	prostate-specific antigen
PT (INR)	prothrombin time
PTH	parathyroid hormone
PTT	partial thromboplastin time
PUFA	polyunsaturated fatty acids
PYY	peptide tyrosine-tyrosine
Q0	extrarenal elimination fraction
qd	every day
QID	four times a day (L: quater in die)
RAEs	retinol activity equivalents
RBC	red blood cell
RCI	recovery from critical illness
RCT	randomized controlled trials
RDA	recommended dietary allowance
RE	retinol equivalents
REE	resting energy expenditure
RFC	reduced folate carrier
RMR	resting metabolic rate
RNA	ribonucleic acid
RRT	renal replacement therapy
RQ	respiratory quotient

RYGB	Roux-en-Y gastric bypass
[S]	serum
SAMe	S-adenosylmethionine
sBP	systolic blood pressure
SBS	shaken baby syndrome
SCFA	short-chain fatty acid
Se	selenium
SG	sleeve gastrectomy
SGIT	sleeve gastrectomy with ileal transposition
SGOT	serum glutamic oxaloacetic transaminase
SGPT	serum glutamic pyruvic transaminase
SIGN	Scottish Intercollegiate Guidelines Network
SIRS	systemic inflammatory response syndrome
SNRIs	serotonin-norepinephrine reuptake inhibitor
SOD	superoxide dismutase
SPN	supplemental parenteral nutrition
SSRIs	selective serotonin reuptake inhibitor
T	trauma
T3	triiodothyronine
T4	thyroxine
T2DM	type 2 diabetes mellitus
TEE	total energy expenditure
TF	tube-feed
TG	triglycerides
THF	tetrahydrofolate

TIBC	total iron-binding capacity
TID	three times a day
TLC	triple-lumen catheter
TLC	therapeutic lifestyle changes
Tmax	maximum body temperature in centigrade
TN	trade name
TNF alpha	tumor necrosis factor alpha
TNU	total urinary nitrogen
TOS	the obesity society
TPA/tPA	tissue plasminogen activator.
TPN	total parenteral nutrition
TSH	thyroid function test
TUL	tolerable upper intake level
UL	upper intake level
USDA	United States Department of Agriculture
UUN	urinary urea nitrogen
UV	ultraviolet
VBG	vertical banded gastroplasty
VCO_2	volume of carbon dioxide
Ve	expired minute ventilation
VLDL	very low density lipoprotein
VO_2	volume of oxygen consumed
WC	waist circumference
Wt	weight
y	year
YY	type of peptide
zn	zink

13.6 Useful Addresses/Websites

American Society for Nutrition
http://www.nutrition.org/

Harvard School of Public Health
http://www.hsph.harvard.edu/nutritionsource/

National Health and Medical Research Council
http://www.nhmrc.gov.au/

healthfinder.gov/
http://healthfinder.gov/

American Nutrition Association
http://americannutritionassociation.org/

National Institute for Clinical Excellence (NICE)
http://www.nice.org.uk/

British Association for Parenteral and Enteral Nutrition (BAPEN)
http://www.bapen.org.uk/

The European Nutrition for Health alliance
http://www.european-nutrition.org/

The European Society for Clinical Nutrition and Metabolism
http://www.espen.org/

The British Dietetic Association
http://www.bda.uk.com/

Australasian College of Nutritional & Environmental Medicine
http://www.acnem.org/modules/mastop_publish/

Trade name = bold   *Drug name = italic*

Trade name = **bold**   Drug name = *italic*

yes

Trade name = bold   Drug name = italic

Trade name = **bold**   Drug name = *italic*

Notes

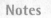

Notes